FEAR KNOCKED
It Was Alzheimer's

The Story of One Man. His Determination.
And the Diagnosis That Made Him Vulnerable.

Lessons Learned From an Advocate Daughter.

Jacqueline Sullivan Wyco

PRAISE FOR *FEAR KNOCKED*

This heart-wrenching debut memoir recounts the life of Wyco's father, John Sullivan—her childhood hero, a pillar in their Boston community, firefighter, and retired Marine. Wyco delves into John's upbringing and early romance with her mother, Beverly; their marriage and her mother's devastating death; John's later remarriage to Marie; and his diagnosis of Alzheimer's at age 74. From the early warning signs that went unheeded to the emotional impact of a debilitating disease to the legal processes involved in caring for an ailing parent, Wyco provides readers with a vulnerable, touching account of "a great man and a good person," as well as a practical guide to navigating the life-altering waters of dementia.

    Wyco's unflinching love for her father is the heart of her writing, reflected in the candid photographs she shares throughout. She contemplates her own childhood and the many lessons her father instilled in her and her brother, John, expressing both her pride in being his daughter and her endless grief—at losing both of her parents and in watching the gradual decline of her father's health. She also chronicles the complicated nature of caregiving, including advocating for her father's needs, navigating medical appointments and treatment, understanding legal ramifications, and making the tough choices that come with end-of-life moments. Her narrative is both pragmatic and evocative, educating readers on real-world issues like identifying the signs of caregiver abuse while offering an intense exploration of the despair that comes with watching a parent approach their last days.

    As Wyco walks the fine line of attempting to abide by her father's wishes and keeping the peace with Marie, she learns valuable lessons for readers who may find themselves in similar situations. This firsthand account of fighting for a loved one's rights in their final days is a moving tribute and an insightful resource for caregivers, family members, and medical advocates.

—Publishers Weekly

"Ms. Wyco's deeply personal yet practical chapter on protecting those with Alzheimer's from financial exploitation demonstrates her commitment to preventing elder abuse through education and advocacy. Her detailed, actionable steps for securing finances and monitoring accounts reflect hard-won wisdom that will prove invaluable to families navigating similar challenges. I particularly appreciate how she emphasizes the importance of early intervention and strategic involvement of professionals like social workers and bank managers to create multiple layers of protection. This chapter alone makes her book an essential resource for families, caregivers, and professionals working to protect our most vulnerable elderly from financial predators."
—*Michael Hackard —Attorney and Founder of Hackard Law, Elder Financial Abuse Expert, and Author.*

"This story redefines the perception of 'vulnerable adults'. Advance directives can be compromised. This book encourages you to be vigilant and teaches you how to regain your loved one's wishes when safeguards fail."
—*Kathleen Welcome—An AmeriCorps Victim Assistance Program member BS in Human Services.*

"This is an inspiring story of an incredible man who lived a life of service to others as a Boston firefighter, father, widow, husband, and friend. It highlights his struggles with end-of-life care in the midst of Alzheimer's and describes his loving daughter's challenges while caring for her father."
—*Mike Keefe—A friend can't describe Mike's relationship with Jack. They were connected on a level that was deeper than friendship.*

"I was angry, reading about the injustices and frustrations! Then I was sad to read what happened in the hospice home. There is no way Jack should have suffered in that way. Unfortunately, coercion and manipulation were set in by the time his daughter Jacqueline realized what was going on. Your first instinct is to think well of people, especially ones that you love and have known for 20 years! I would have enjoyed meeting Jack. He sounds amazing. This book will tap into readers' emotions that will linger long after the book is read, as they have for me."
—*Celia Hartigan—RN.*

"The beautiful love and relationship of a daughter and her dad. Right to the very end. I found myself tearful several times, happy tears as well as sad. I also found myself reliving some of the crazy times in the city growing up. The areas Jacqueline speaks of were my stomping grounds. From where I lived, to where I went to school. Then being married with 2 of my 4 children, number 3 was on the way during the layoffs. Living through the series of arson fires, I knew some of those involved. It was a walk down memory lane. I felt Jacqueline's love, pain, her father's pride, and hers for him. What an incredible man he was. I only knew him as the firefighter he was in padding. What he was put through during this Alzheimer's process was cruel. Coercive control is a form of elder abuse but not enough is known. A wise woman once said to me, 'You're not responsible for what you don't know but once you do, then it's your responsibility to attempt to change or fix it.' To this day, Jacqueline is attempting to right an unbelievably broken system. The lessons learned were profound."

—Kathy Minehan—Co-Leader WINGS CISM Team, Massachusetts. Kathy's husband, Lieutenant Stephen Minehan, of the Boston Fire Department, died in a nine-alarm fire in a warehouse on the Charlestown Pier while working to save his fellow firefighters on June 24, 1994. For the past 30 years, Kathy has been dedicated to helping thousands of grieving widows in need of grief support.

"Such an intense and loving tribute. Jacqueline's parents were salt-of-thee-arth people, and so is she. This book is full of practical tips for the power of attorney and health care proxy. Other families dealing with Alzheimer's will learn from her experience."

—Sue Barron—A decades-long Spinning Instructor, Certified Fitness Trainer, and Sports Nutritionist, who's experienced Alzheimer's in her own family.

"*Fear Knocked* is a riveting, powerful, and evocative story of life in Boston in the 1970s and 1980s. Written in a pungent, direct, eloquent yet incredibly moving style. Jacqueline teaches her readers by what she learned through the treachery and betrayal of a woman who took advantage of her father's declining judgment. This story is an extraordinary testament to an amazing man, her childhood, her mother's strength and courage, and her parents' undying love. Jacqueline's father had grit and determination, and he honored his wife's memory with an extraordinary and perilous cross-country ride. He was selfless in his dedication to family."

—*Hayden A. Duggan, Ed.D.*—
President and Founder of the On-Site Academy, Gardner, MA.,
Team Clinician for the Boston Police Stress Support Unit CISM Team,
Chief Psychologist for Boston EMS Peer Support Team.
Licensed Clinical Psychologist,
Doctorate Clinical Psychology and Public Practice from
Harvard Graduate School of Education.
Designated Forensic Psychologist (inactive)
in the Commonwealth of Massachusetts.
Instructor for the International Critical Incident Stress Foundation,
Adjunct Professor for Anna Maria College in Paxton, Massachusetts,
and Author.

Copyright 2024 by Jacqueline Sullivan Wyco
All rights reserved. Published and printed in the USA 2025.

No part of this book may be quoted without express written permission of the publisher, except for editorial reviews limited to 400 words.

ISBN paperback: 979-8-218-83022-9
ISBN ebook (print replica): 979-8-218-64361-4
ISBN ebook (reflowable): 979-8-9947058-0-3

HEA039140 HEALTH & FITNESS / Diseases & Conditions/ Alzheimer& Dementia
FAM001020 FAMILY & RELATIONSHIPS / Abuse / Elder Abuse
BIO036000 BIOGRAPHY & AUTOBIOGRAPHY / Fire & Emergency Services

https://jacquelinesullivanwyco.com/

DENBURG PRESS, LLC
PO Box 163, Venice FL 34284

Editor: Mark Mathes. mmathes1@gmail.com
Book cover design and interior formatting: Nancy R. Koucky. https://nrkdesigns.com/

This book Created by Humans.

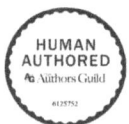

FEAR KNOCKED
It Was Alzheimer's

The Story of One Man. His Determination.
And the Diagnosis That Made Him Vulnerable.

Lessons Learned From an Advocate Daughter.

Jacqueline Sullivan Wyco

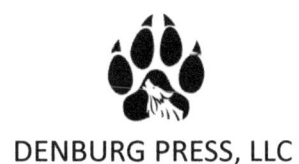

DENBURG PRESS, LLC

Contact the publisher for quantity discounts of this book for your book club or organization.
The author appreciates reviews at online book sites, including Amazon and Goodreads.

Share your comments and stay updated with future developments.
Contact the author at jswforu@gmail.com

Follow Jacqueline on LinkedIn.
https://www.linkedin.com/in/jacqueline-sullivan-wyco-43153528/

༄༅༄༅༄༅

Disclosure

This book is based on the author's personal experiences and her research on Alzheimer's. The author's goal is to educate her readers. The content is true and presented from the author's perspective. References include but are not limited to her father's medical and financial documents, legal and social work counsel and email correspondences, psychology journals, and medical research. To maintain the privacy and anonymity of some professionals and family members their names have been changed. Details such as physical properties and places of residence have been generalized to protect the privacy of the family and friends portrayed in this book.

Dedication

For more than 50 years, I witnessed my father's resilience and strength. Through crises and chaos, he stayed calm and focused. He was methodical. The life lessons I received from my father were invaluable. As a father, he was exceptional, but his drive to help others made him a special human being.

My book is dedicated to my father.

Contents

Chapter 1	About My Father	1
Chapter 2	Imprints from My Childhood	13
Chapter 3	Love and Loss	28
Chapter 4	Transformation	33
Chapter 5	Alzheimer's, The Warning Signs	42
Chapter 6	The Progression	51
Chapter 7	Why the Sudden Change of Heart?	62
Chapter 8	First Came Alzheimer's, Then Came Marriage	67
Chapter 9	Things Aren't Always What They Appear	75
Chapter 10	A Fragile State Teetering on Volatile	80
Chapter 11	The Opposition	89
Chapter 12	The Ultimatum	108
Chapter 13	Optical Illusion	116
Chapter 14	Proof Wasn't Enough	122
Chapter 15	In the Eyes of Judgment	129
Chapter 16	Patterns Emerge	142
Chapter 17	By Willful Omission	146
Chapter 18	The Quest for Guardianship	153
Chapter 19	Hospice: Their Mission vs. Their Capability	159
Chapter 20	The Struggle to Maintain Peace	165

Chapter 21	Nearing the End	171
Chapter 22	Pain Out of Control	180
Chapter 23	The Window	185
Chapter 24	Unfathomable	191
Chapter 25	Letting Go	198
Chapter 26	Tribute	204
Chapter 27	Life After	213
Chapter 28	Empty Promises	220
Chapter 29	Healing	227
Chapter 30	Advocates and Advanced Directives	232
Chapter 31	Guardianship	239
Chapter 32	Why Lucidity Is Important	241
Chapter 33	Types of Abuse	244
Chapter 34	How to Protect Against Financial Exploitation	248
Obituary		259
Endnotes		262
Bibliography		271
Acknowledgments		275
Author's Note		277
About the Author		279

Fear knocked on the door.
Faith answered.
And there was no one there.

—Old Irish proverb

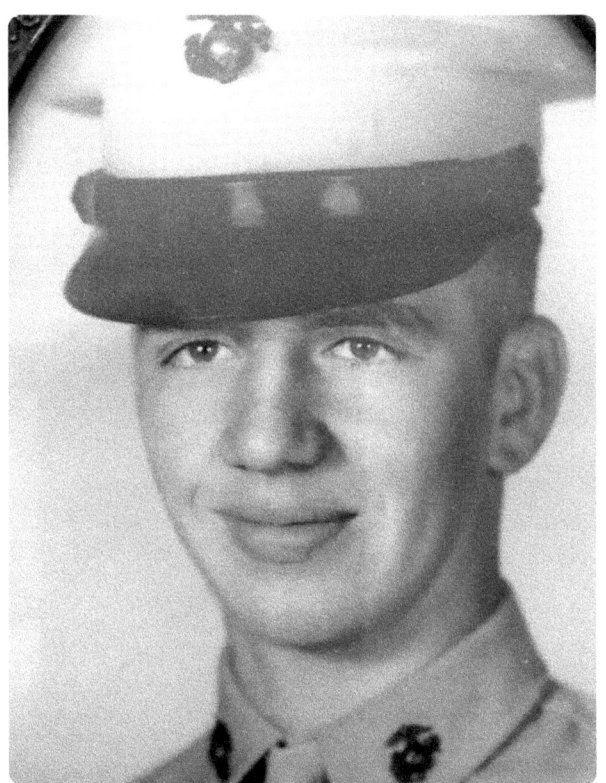
John Sullivan, US Marine Corps (1956-1958)
From the Sullivan Family Collection

Chapter 1
About My Father

To hear my firefighter father tell me he had Alzheimer's is something I would have never predicted. He never asked, "Why me?" Even though, he lived in a mind that betrayed him every day, during his last seven years. It was a battle he couldn't win. He thought his end was far away, yet it was closer than he ever envisioned. There was a fear in his eyes that I hadn't seen before. He grew lost in places where he once knew and stumbled to find the right words to say. I caught glimpses of the awkward stares and heard whispers as he walked into a room. They did not know the hell he lived in, for he wore a smile for all to see, while tears wept silently inside. My father was a man living with a disease in which he had no control. Alzheimer's took charge and changed his existence.

The Early Years

Both my father's parents immigrated from County Cork, Ireland. My grandfather, John Sullivan, was a farmer and a quiet giant of a man. He arrived in the United States in 1922 and hauled freight as a longshoreman on Boston's docks. My grandmother came to Boston in 1927. She cleaned houses as many Irish women did at that time. They couldn't get over the fact that they had never met before migrating to the United States. She and my grandfather were seven years apart in age. Boston's neighborhood of Jamaica Plain became their home after they married in 1928. One year later, in August 1929, the Great Depression began. It lasted for ten years and during this time their four girls were born, and one died. Becoming unemployed was a fear that everyone had, and my grandparents' three young children were all very close in age. The stock market crashed, banks closed and economic panic set in. "This was the longest and deepest downturn in the history of the United States and the modern industrial economy."[1] On March 5, 1939, my grandparents' only son, John J. Sullivan Jr. was born. My father was five days shy of six months old when World War II began, and the Depression ended.

My father was taller than other grade school kids his age. He was always on the move. Back then, there was no ADHD diagnosis. One nun at school understood him. Instead of homework, she gave him tasks. His assignment became catching tadpoles for the class to observe a frog's growth. However, not every teacher saw what he needed or took the time to figure out how to redirect his restlessness and excess energy. When he grew intolerable in other teachers' classes, they punished him.

One nun had a signature trademark punishment.

My father said, "Sister Mary, I'll never forget her. She used to have a tall jar with these long *rat's hands* soaking in vinegar on her desk." Rat's hands, he said, were like a thin strong bamboo-like reed.

He said, "She'd call me up to the front of the class, pull one out, open my palm, and whack me on the hand until the skin opened. It felt like paper cuts. They stung to the high heavens."

But nothing she did could curb his rambunctious behavior. Although she tried, she never broke him. He was a spirit who couldn't be contained.

During his eighth-grade year, he went to his father and told him he wanted to quit school. His father didn't yell or talk him out of it. Instead, his father told him what his reality would become if he quit.

He said, "If you do, you will work hard for the rest of your life."

That didn't faze my father. He quit and never looked back. At thirteen years old he earned ten cents a day in a yarn factory, a workplace that would be closed by OSHA's standards today. In the summer, the temperature in the brick factory multiplied to what it was outside.

My father said, "Oh, that place, it was god-awful. It was like a dungeon."

A permanent haze covered the windows and his only view to the outside was where the sun found its way through the dried-out cracks in the walls. There were no fans, no AC, no ventilation whatsoever. Fibers from the loom machines hung in the air and clung to his sweat. Then the day came, like school, when enough was enough. From a young age, he lived life on his own terms. He went to work as a laborer for his uncle. He mixed, wheelbarrowed, and shoveled concrete all day long. Even though he loved it, he was searching for something more.

My father made a commitment the day he enlisted. *Once a Marine, always a Marine*, wasn't just a motto. What it meant to be a Marine lived within my father for the rest of his life. My father was stationed for two years at Camp Lejeune, NC. He rarely talked about the details of his time in the service. Rather, he spoke more about the Marines in general. He was proud to serve as a Marine. It gave him a foundation and shaped him into the man he became.

My mother, Beverly Penna, fell in love with my father and married him soon after he returned home. She grew up with her older brother, in the post-depression housing development, or the Project as it was called, adjacent to my father's home on Round Hill Street. Their mother separated from their father and traveled to the Jamaica Plain neighborhood of Boston from Philadelphia, Pennsylvania in 1946. Her mother signed up for welfare when they arrived. Something that she didn't want to do but had to do until she secured a job. She was a nursing assistant at Peter Bent Brigham Hospital in Boston.

My father was seven and in the first grade at Blessed Sacrament, the same school my mother attended. When you're five and seven, a two-year age difference is significant. They weren't friends, but they knew each other by sight. Mainly Irish Catholics lived in their neighborhood and my mother stuck out among the fair-skinned, blue-eyed, freckled faces with her dark olive complexion and mahogany brown eyes. Kids picked on her and made fun of her long skinny legs. My mother felt insecure because she was always taller than the other girls. She tried not to be noticed.

When my father came home from the Marines, my mother was introduced to him by a friend they had in common. At seventeen, my mother looked much older than she was. Underneath my mother's long jet-black hair, tall stature, and striking beauty was the confidence of a woman ahead of her time. It was 1958 and my father's parents weren't pleased about my father's decision to marry. However, my father was of age and eventually, they saw the woman he fell in love with.

After my parents were married, they lived in a small apartment in Roslindale, a neighborhood near the West Roxbury border of Boston. My mother worked full-time as an operator for the New England Telephone Company, and my father joined the Boston Plasterers and Cement Mason's Union. They cleaned banks and offices at night to achieve their goal of owning a home.

Boston was my father's backyard, and he loved it as much as he loved cement finishing. The harder he worked, the greater satisfaction he felt. For thirty-five years, he worked in Local 534. He used to joke and say that Boston was his city because he helped build it. He worked round the clock, sometimes finishing concrete. It's a job that can't be rushed. Floating concrete starts when it stiffens and depending on the weather, the temperature outside, and the additives used, concrete could take hours before it was ready to bull float and level out. There was an art to what he did. Working the slab too soon could cause the concrete to weaken and crack. If it dried out too much before it was trawled and finished, the slab was prone to pitting and deteriorating quickly. His finish work was impeccable, he was a perfectionist.

You name the modern Boston structure, and he most likely helped build it. In 1960 construction began on the Prudential Tower. By completion in 1964, it would be the tenth tallest building in the world and the tallest in North America. Fifty-two stories above the pavement, nothing but the weather conditions surrounded him. He didn't like heights, but adjusted and overcame his fears, like most things in his life.

In his early twenties, he had developed a reputation on the job. Many knew him and liked him. Others who didn't know him recognized him by sight. He had a mustache, long sideburns, and a thick head of light brown hair. He swooped it back on the top and then combed the sides to meet at the nape of his neck. In the late fall, he wore a scally. When it was colder, he tucked it under a knit cap neatly folded up on all sides above his ears.

He had built himself a good life. He seemed to have it all. But his strengths sometimes converged with his greatest weakness. Alcohol dragged him down and took him out on many a night. A side of him surfaced that even he didn't know after a few drinks. He tore up bars, and never, ever walked away from a fight he didn't start. One night, a group of guys in a pool room tested my father. They purposefully egged him on, walked behind him, and bumped into his pool stick while he tried to make a shot. Without an *excuse me*, or a *sorry pal* after the third time, my father turned around. In his Boston accent, he said, "Hey! You know you bumped into me."

Then three surrounded him. My father didn't back down. They clubbed him in the head with the butts of their sticks. My father had a personal code. He fought fair, and he used his fists. He needed nothing else. His fingers were long, and his hands were always rough and calloused. When he told the story, he put his hands on his head and said, "Boy, that hurt bad. But I kept swinging, and I knocked all three out."

Another barroom banned him after he blacked out and waged a war on the wall-to-wall mirror behind the bartender.

My father said, "I liked the sound of breaking glass when I had a few. I don't remember, but I shattered the mirror with my beer bottles."

When he walked in the next day, the bartender said, "Sully, what are you doing here? You can't be in here. You destroyed the place last night."

My father had blacked out and the string of nights he didn't make it home for supper added up to weeks, then months, and years. Booze exerted power over him. This wasn't what my mother envisioned for their marriage. And regardless of how many times my father promised to stop drinking after an argument, he'd start again. He couldn't kick it. So, my mother kicked him out. She told him, if he stopped drinking for good, he could come home. It was tough love. He needed to find his way.

In 1971, my father embraced sobriety and never drank again. A clearer, more defined sense of himself emerged. He asked God to grant him serenity, and he prayed to accept the things he could not change, the courage to change the things he could, and the wisdom to know the difference. My father kneeled by the side of their bed, clasped his hands, and bowed his head, every night, before he went to sleep and said this prayer. It sat on his dresser in a frame, underneath my mother's picture on the wall.

Fear Knocked — Jacqueline Sullivan Wyco

In the summer of 1972, I was seven years old and unaware of how close we were to losing my mother. Early on while carrying my brother, her doctors discovered cancer. By the ninth month, the tumor grew to the size of a basketball. It spread and attached itself to her organs, like an octopus. The surgery she needed was called a Whipple. They scheduled the delivery on December 11, 1972, by caesarian section. The doctor's plan was for her to come home after the birth to regain her strength for the surgery.

Meanwhile, my father decided to rip out our kitchen, down to the studs. Plastic sheeting and blankets covered the holes for the vinyl sliding windows on order. The frigid air blew through the cracks between the studs and the boarded frame. This wasn't ideal for coming home with a new infant. My father insulated the walls as fast as he could. I think this was my father's way of moving forward. He planned a future with my mother and that's what he focused on.

This surgery would be tough, not only for my mother, but also for her doctors. It took about six to eight weeks before she went back in for the surgery. I had to stay at a neighbor's house after school and my father's mother cared for my brother. He was working at a new job site at the Faulkner Hospital, finishing concrete for their new parking garage. My mother's room was at the back of the hospital where she could see the construction. My father wore an orange shirt so she could easily spot him. I don't know if the union placed him there because they knew my mother was a patient there, or if it was by coincidence. Seeing my father every day was significant to her. It helped her heal. I realized how much when I found his shirt years later, neatly folded in her drawer.

I wasn't allowed to visit my mother inside the hospital, and my father knew how much I was missing her. He brought me up one day after work and had me wait on the patients' back deck of the hospital. When she came out and saw me, she hugged me tight. I was lonesome without her. She understood and told me, not to worry, she'd be home soon. Every night my father made me supper. He mostly boiled hot dogs, and opened a can of beans, adding maple syrup to make them taste better. I don't remember much else he cooked. I only remember the empty feeling of my mother not being home.

The two surgeons took part of my mother's small intestine, large intestine, part of her pancreas, and her entire spleen. When she returned home, she was in rough shape. She was weak and lost so much weight that the pressure of sitting in a chair caused her pain. At almost eight years old, I learned how to cook, change diapers, feed, and care for my baby brother. My mother needed to rest and when she went to lie down, my father gave her a bell to ring when she needed him. I heard her scream, *Sully*, one night after supper, from their upstairs bedroom. She sounded frantic as she rang the bell. I yelled to my father when I heard her. He jumped up the stairs two at a time to help my mother. The pain was so severe, she couldn't get up by herself to reach the bathroom.

To survive pancreatic cancer without chemo or radiation in 1972 defied medical logic. Yet, she did. Cancer couldn't compete with her warrior spirit. Her resolve mirrored that of my father's. Each day she grew stronger. For both of my parents, staying present, one day at a time, strengthened their focus. My father stayed sober, and my mother beat the odds and survived. They were joined by marriage and were bonded through the trials they came up against.

In the early 1970s, the Boston building boom faded and guys on the job moved out of state to places like Oklahoma where construction work was in demand. One of the finishers, a close friend of my father's, moved to Alaska and worked on the oil pipeline. Others stayed, took certification tests, and changed careers like my father. A friend of his stopped by one afternoon and gave my father an application for the fire department, which he had no intention of taking. But my mother encouraged him. She saw the job offered stability, and in 1973, my father became a Boston firefighter. It wasn't in his blood. It wasn't a long-held dream of his. He did it because he had a family to take care of.

My father was first stationed in Brighton, at Oak Square, a small community eight miles on the outskirts of downtown Boston. The firehouse sat on the opposite side of a traffic rotary with century-old oak trees. Not many emergency runs and very few fires made for long days and even longer nights. There's nothing my father loathed more than sitting idle waiting to work. Yet, standing by is part of a firefighter's profession. He wanted to be in the action, and he put in a transfer to Ladder 7 Meetinghouse Hill in Dorchester. The firehouse sat high on the hill with the First Parish Church and North America's oldest public elementary school, the Mather School[2], across from them on a dead end. By the time my father transferred, the streets had turned into an all-out untamed modern version of the Wild West.

The city of Boston in the 1970s was in crisis mode. There was crime, arson, and drugs galore. Neighborhood streets were percolating with unrest from desegregation busing, also known as integration busing, or busing as my parents called it. Protests emerged, and the violence bled into the streets and spawned a hatred that no one anticipated. "In 1974, the US District Court ordered the desegregation of public schools."[3] [From the Desegregation Busing Encyclopedia Boston.] And institutions of learning from the oldest in the education system to the newly constructed schools became the hub of prejudice and hostility. Rage-driven students vandalized neighborhood schools from block to block from the inside out. The public schools in Boston, including where I lived in West Roxbury, and in Dorchester, where my father worked, became the symbols of an era marked by bitter division.

Dorchester in the 1970s, had fallen into the grips of pimps, crackheads, dealers, and thieves. Crime infested its 6 square miles. You needed eyes in the back of your head driving through the neighborhood. And there were streets you didn't dare cross. But my father had no choice. He had to get to work. Gunfire during the daylight hours in Dorchester was common. Bullets came close to his truck one day just after he passed Franklin Park Zoo. On another day, on his way home, going through Jamaica Plain the neighborhood that borderedDorchester, a body lay near Lemuel Shattuck, a psychiatric hospital with a less-than-stellar reputation back then over on Morton Street. He barely stopped at the red lights, just enough to see if anyone was coming, and then he drove right through. The firehouse was so busy that many times he had to jump on the ladder truck before he could change into his uniform.

As darkness approached, air horn blasts, howls, and yelps, from fire, police, and ambulance sirens consumed the air. Gangs roamed the area. Many were doped up and strung out, some were as high as kites. Rivals fought and marked their territory. Some members turned on each other. But these weren't the only groups who residents feared. Others roamed aimlessly, just looking for an opportunity. Guns and knives were easy to get, but nothing was off-limits to threaten, maim, or kill. Smashing car windows with bricks and robbing people at traffic signals was how some earned their living.

On Fridays, my father's check came in after lunch at the station. Usually, he worked concrete during the weekdays. He paid guys for his day tours so he could work the second job. The fire department didn't pay enough to support a family of four. My father's schedule rotated, and between the two jobs, he worked six or seven days with two-night tours minimum each week. My mother filled my father's role during his absence. She protected, cared for, and provided for all our needs, and I felt as safe with her as I did with him.

On Fridays after school, my mother took my brother and me to the firehouse to pick up his check. My brother sat in the back seat of our gold-colored 1969 Olds Cutlass wagon, and I sat in the front. Back then, we didn't wear seatbelts, and everything was manually operated except for the rear window in the tailgate door. My mother had a ritual. She tucked her pocketbook under my seat, then she popped in an eight-track tape of Barbara Streisand or Johnny Mathis for the ride. She kept a butcher's meat hook under the front driver's seat. The short, curved sharp hook with a wooden handle fit snugly in the palm of a hand against the knuckles. She had no qualms about reaching for it and using it if she had to. When we got to the Franklin Park Zoo traffic light, my mother gripped both hands on the wheel and she turned on high alert.

It didn't matter how hot it was, we had to roll up our window and push down the lock on our door. It was non-negotiable. She didn't have to tell us we were about to go down Columbia Road. If the light was green, she hit the gas. If we were approaching a yellow with no car in front of us, she doubled down, and her foot stomped to the floor. She rarely hit the brakes. But getting caught at a red light came with a rule. My father said, "Leave enough room between you and the car in front, in case there's an ambush and you need to get away."

Certain lights were notorious for smash and grabs. He said, "If you're the first car, stop, then go through. Don't wait for the green."

My mother's head swiveled like an owl. She looked one way, then the other, in front, behind, and to the sides. If we got stopped by the cops, my father told her, "Just tell them, your husband is on the Fire Ladder 7 and you're on your way there to pick up his check."

I remember seeing neighborhoods plagued with addicts. Crack, heroin, speed, and other drugs slowly sucked the life out of the residents and their communities. It was a public health catastrophe on steroids. All along Columbia Road in Dorchester, the homeless pushed shopping carts with garbage bags filled with bottles and cans that they dug out of the trash barrels. They were focused and determined to get every cent they could, but no amount of nickel redemptions was enough to escape. And no one was coming to rescue them.

Many picked through the Salvation Army bins that had clothes half hanging out the chute and donated bags stacked to the side. They wore layers of clothing. When it got too hot, oversized crud-stained winter coats hung over the sides. Some had sleeping bags. They were shoved in front of their carts. Everything they owned they pushed in their cart and everything they owned told the story of what it was like to live on the street.

Some sat on street corners, and others propped themselves up against the newspaper vending machines. Several yelled at cars and those who passed by. Others exposed themselves to hallucinogenic realms and altered states. They stood on sidewalks, in front of liquor stores, and hung out on street corners. Some talked to the sky and argued out loud with a person who didn't exist.

On this day, we had to take Geneva Ave., the side street and the residential neighborhood of the infamous double stabbings, shootings, and murders. All of which could take place in one day. We took a left turn onto it to get to the firehouse.

McDonald's, and Burger King paper bags, cups, and empty French fry containers flew from cars. People on sidewalks dropped theirs as they finished. Empties rolled down the curb and filled the sewer grates in the street. Ethnic corner markets had accordion-style iron gates pushed to one side with a padlock attached. The first-floor apartments of three-story homes featured bars on the front door and windows all around.

Kids of all ages spray painted property. They were free to express how they felt. I saw teenagers walking with bats. Some used them as protection, and others used them to attack. I was thirteen, and these kids were my age. They were hardened by life in the city. They were groomed for a life on the street by those only a couple of years older than them.

The bigger the boom box, the more attention it drew. They were carried on top of one shoulder or were rested at a corner against a building. The vibration throbbed through the car and into my chest as we drove by. I saw pit bulls wearing monstrous spiked collars. Drug dealers made them vicious. Dogs were trained to attack. Instilling fear in others made them feel powerful. I watched crowds of people part as they walked down the sidewalk.

Pedestrians were sometimes part of a scheme to rob or carjack drivers. Thugs slowly strutted across the street in front of cars and stared down drivers to slow down. My mother didn't flinch. She drove at one speed. *Fast*, and they moved out of her way. She weaved through the street like a race car in the Indy 500. She dodged them and others who crossed. When double-parked cars and delivery trucks blocked the lane, she drove on the opposite side of the road. When oncoming drivers played chicken, more often than not, they were the ones who pulled to the side.

The stop sign at the end of the avenue signaled we were close. On the right, we passed Saint Peter's Church and the dilapidated Victorian behind it up on the hill, from the TV show, *This Old House*. That's when the tension eased. We reached the home stretch. Two seconds to go and we'd arrive to pick up my father's check.

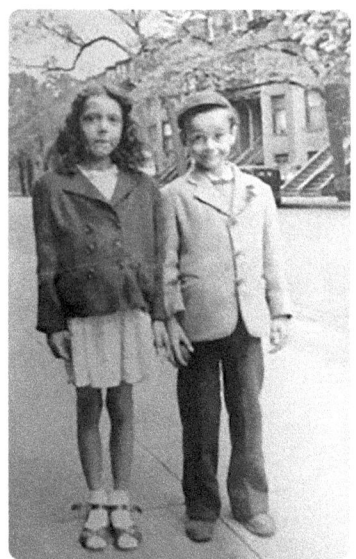

Beverly Penna ("Sis", the nickname given to her by her brother Joel) and her brother Joel in Boston.
Sullivan Family Photo Collection

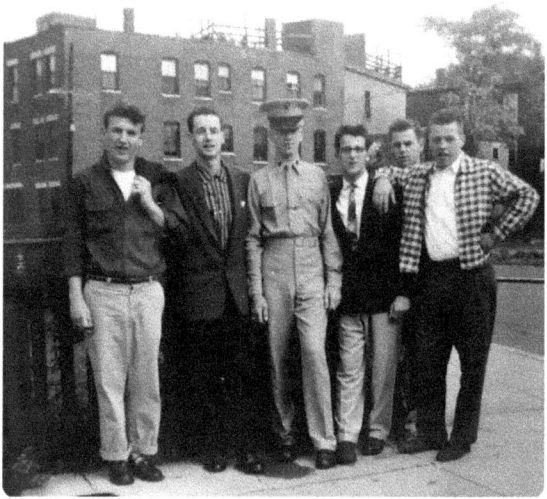

Marine John Sullivan (third from the left) in front of his home with his buddies on Round Hill Street, Jamaica Plain. The project behind him is where Beverly and her brother lived.
From the Sullivan Family Photo Collection

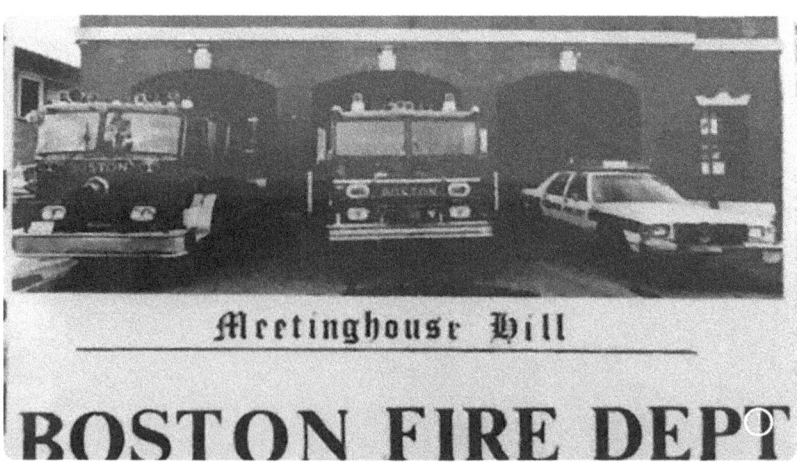

Boston Fire Department Ladder Seven Engine 17
Printed with verbal permission from the Boston Fire Department

Chapter 2
Imprints From My Childhood

I always felt safe with my father as a child and growing up through my teenage years. He walked with purpose, in a way that others could read he was no one to tangle with. He stood tall at six foot four. He looked rugged and weathered. My father showed me how to carry myself and keep trouble at a distance without realizing it.

When my father was home, he usually spent time on a project, or a hobby, and he always invited me to help him. When we planted a garden together, he just didn't plop in the plants. He told me where to dig, how far apart to space them, how to fertilize them, and when to water them. He told me the why behind everything. At five and six years old, I understood what it meant to be compassionate. At about the age of nine, I remember picking vegetables down behind our garage where he planted his garden. My father took my mother's laundry basket, filled it to the top with vegetables, and brought me with him to the Children's Home for Little Wanderers, an orphanage in Boston close to our home. I remember walking into the building and the smile on the lady's face when she saw the softball-sized beefsteak tomatoes and giant cucumbers. That same year before Christmas, he and my mother decided they wanted to bring a couple of children home from the same orphanage for the holiday. When he went to talk with the administrator, she said they stopped allowing it because the kids were so upset when they had to return. I knew what it was like to have, and my mother and father taught me to give.

Motivation was an ever-evolving state for my father. It's something he worked on. His inspiration came from many places. He read the Boston Globe, from front to back when he was home. A good quote never went to waste. Back then the Boston Globe published a reflection for the day quotation. If one inspired him, he'd cut it out, and hang it up, in the corner of a mirror, a frame, the fridge, or at the table. You never knew when a new quote would pop up. Like this one, by Elbert Hubbard, which he stuck in the corner of a picture near the back door. *One machine can do the work of fifty ordinary men. No machine can do the work of one extraordinary man.*

Then there were the obituaries. He read them just like he did the sports section. On his rare day off, he'd lay on the couch with his feet up sideways, watching a ball game, or the news. From the living room, he'd yell out to my mother in the kitchen while she cooked. He talked fast when he wanted her attention. In his deep voice, he called my mother Sis, her childhood nickname given to her by her brother. They'd reminisce about the person who died and the neighborhood, then he'd go back and read some more. But obits didn't have to be someone he knew for him to engage my mother again. He studied regular people and their history. Their accomplishments intrigued him, especially when he learned how they started in life.

I saw how he attuned himself to his environment when we were out. He took notice of those who had fallen out of society's norms. The economic downturn during the 1970s was closely linked to increasing homelessness in the city. One day, my father and I were walking under the bridge that crossed into Haymarket from the North End. A homeless man prone in a gutter asked for change. My ears were stinging from the cold. The man, probably only in his fifties, barely had enough energy to raise his head off the pavement to ask for money. I heard him ask, but I ignored him and walked by. I looked back when I realized my father had stopped. He put his hand into his pocket and gave him a couple of bucks.

In a low and gentle tone, my father said, "Here you go, pal."

I said, "Dad, why did you do that? He's just going to go buy a bottle."

He said, "That could be me."

My father had walked the fine line between having everything and losing everything before he gave up drinking. He saw a version of

Imprints From My Childhood

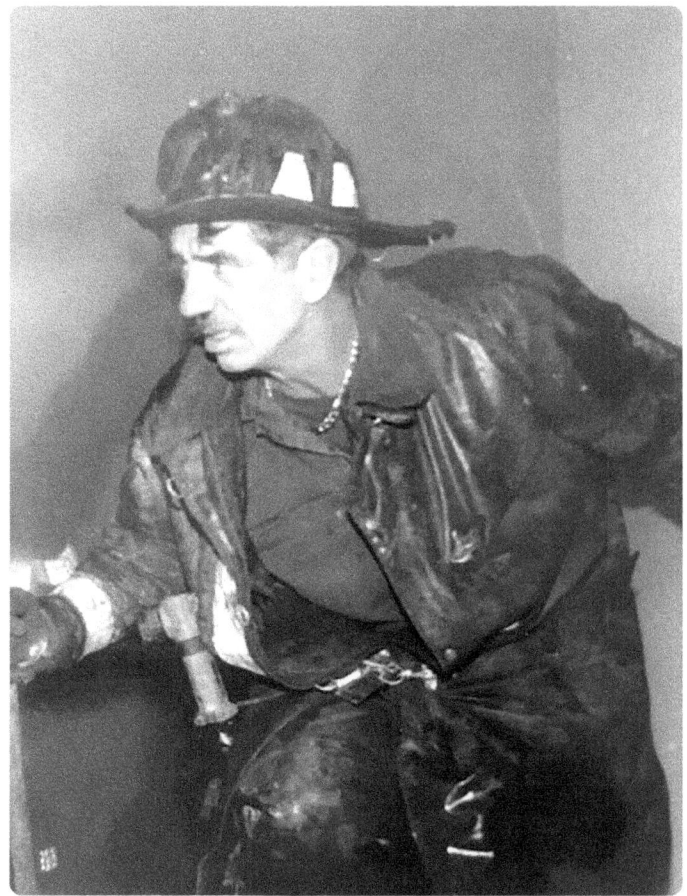

John Sullivan (known by Sully, his nickname on the Fire Department) making his way up a stairway in Dorchester.
From the Sullivan Family photo collection, photographer unknown

Reflection for the day
One machine can do the work of fifty ordinary men. No machine can do the work of one extraordinary man.
ELBERT HUBBARD

Cut out and saved by John from the Boston Globe's Reflection for the Day.
From the Sullivan Family Collection

himself in that man. He understood a man's worth as a human being went beyond his circumstances.

Homelessness and crime were surging during the late 1970s, and the crime-ridden streets of Dorchester collided with an epic wave of arson. "In 1977 Boston was swept up by another arson spree, with almost 100 buildings going up in flames. But while those fires were lit in an attempt to collect insurance premiums, the arson spree of the 1980s was a little more personal," The New York Times reported.[4] From the Grunge online magazine, "The Untold Truth Behind The 1982 Boston Arson Spree."

The Dorchester section of Boston languished in ruins. Abandoned boarded-up three-deckers became crack houses and insurance fraud grew rampant. Some owners burned down their own houses, regardless of who could get hurt. Gasoline-soaked rags and Molotov cocktails turned a fire within seconds into an inferno. They filled sandwich bags with gasoline and placed them above doorways to fall when a firefighter came through the door. Firefighters never knew what they were walking into. Putting out fires and saving lives was their job. They were the humble heroes of this era.

When my father came home, he told us the stories of the fires, the tragic deaths, and the close calls. Before he told stories, he pointed to the kitchen door and said, "Nothing I tell you, leaves this house." And my brother and I knew he meant it. Because behind every tragedy, there was a person. Their lives and what happened on the job weren't to be talked about with our friends or the rest of our family.

He sat in his thick rock maple armchair at the kitchen table sipping his coffee while my mother cooked his bacon and eggs in the cast-iron skillet. As he told the story, he re-enacted the scene. My brother and I were taken on a ride that began when the call came in. He drove the tiller, and he ducked his head as if he were just driving out of the bay. Then he moved his entire body as he explained the ladder truck speeding up, taking turns down the narrow streets with cars parked on both sides. He described the pedestrians running out of the way as the air horn blasted.

He said, "The driver turned the corner, and I couldn't make the swing. Cars were on both sides. I creamed the car on the corner and three after that. I couldn't help it."

He made us feel like we were there. He said, "I saw the smoke two blocks away. The fire was roaring. I jumped off the truck and grabbed the adze." The adze was his favorite tool, similar to an ax. I smelled the smoke and felt the heat as he opened up the roof.

Then there were the car accidents. Some of them were horrific. I'll never forget one call. A man crashed into a pole. It went through his windshield into his chest and through his seat. They had to cut the pole and stabilize it before extracting him from his car in his driver's seat. He was transported to the hospital with the pole attached. After recapping the night's last call, my father's body relaxed. He leaned back with his legs stretched out to the side of the kitchen table and dropped his hands over the arm of his chair. My father appreciated coming home. He said he was lucky to make it out of some of the fires he was in. But I didn't believe it was luck. I thought he was invincible.

The following link is to YouTube from Edison Green Fire on January 29, 1988. Flames broke out on a winter night in a three-decker with multiple family members trapped inside. Here, my father is on the second-floor porch, going back and forth inside the building and lifting one after the other over the railing to his fellow Boston Firefighters. https://www.youtube.com/watch?v=8UXSlzhthO0

⸙⸙⸙

When he came up against a problem, he repeated this quote: *Where there is a will there is a way.* Repetition and positive thinking became the combination that unlocked all possibilities for him. Every problem had a solution and that included a crisis. The trickle-down effect of the oil shortage during the 1970s caused an energy crisis in America and hardship for many blue-collar families. Gas rationing led to many stations running out of fuel, often as vehicles idled in line. The cost of everything skyrocketed. There was panic in the air. And while everyone was wondering how they were going to heat their homes and pay the bills, my father took on his approach to solving the problem.

He had a plan. He ripped out all the radiators on the first floor and left the upstairs ones as a backup to a woodstove he installed himself. My father didn't buy wood. Instead, he searched for trees and harvested firewood from those that were toppled by storms. The number of small forests in and around Boston would surprise you. He researched everything he bought. It always had to be the best. And when he bought a chainsaw, it was no exception. It was a beast. A Jonsered, made in Sweden and built to last.

My father taught himself how to read a tree, where to cut it, and how to predict which way it would fall. He brought home some mammoth-sized logs, some from trees he had to cut up into rounds and roll up an embankment to the truck. I remember the day he stopped me to count the rings on the section closest to the trunk. When he asked me how many I counted, he said that's how old the tree is. It was close to a hundred years old. In his way, he was telling me it was worthy of notice. My father respected all of life, including that of nature.

He cut firewood all spring and summer long to prepare for the cold New England winters. He'd split logs into two-foot lengths with an ax on the nights he was off. Then he used the chisel and a sledgehammer for the massive rounds from the limbs and trunks. After supper, I helped him. When it got closer to dark, my mother flipped on the spotlights that lit up our yard. My father kept track of how much he burned each year, so the following season he'd have a better idea of how much he needed.

Wood by the cord equaled one hundred twenty-eight cubic feet. He'd start the first couple of rows and outline the width and I'd follow and cross-stack the logs. Four feet wide, four feet high, and eight feet long measured a cord. The next section would begin right next to it. Fourteen cords we had lined up on one side of our yard and back down the other. It could be below zero outside in the winter with blizzard conditions and we'd be sweltering inside. And the blizzard of 1978 proved that you can never be too prepared for a nor'easter in New England.

Before computer-generated weather models, meteorologists were notorious for being wrong. Many storms went out to sea, and some fizzled out altogether. Regardless, my parents always were prepared. In the storm, two weeks before the blizzard, we had a record 21-inch snowfall for the area. Some believed the blizzard would be no different from the storm we just shoveled out of. Others thought we might have missed the brunt of it because it didn't start earlier in the afternoon, as forecasted.

My father was on his three nights off and he got a call from a contractor the day before to plow. He immediately said yes. My father never turned down work to make extra money and asked me if I wanted to go with him. He was sent to plow commercial properties. The two that I remember well were the Old Mr. Boston, a distillery on Massachusetts Avenue in Boston, near the well-known Victoria's Diner, and the other was a large housing development in Revere. Late afternoon, about rush hour, the snow fell as much as four inches an hour. The wipers on the truck couldn't keep up with the falling snow. They froze up continually, even with the truck's defroster on high. Often, my father had to stop and scrape the ice off the wipers and the snow from the headlights to see. I watched him through the windshield. He squinted his eyes and steadied himself as the gusts pounded against him and the truck. Within a few seconds, his mustache grew icicles, and his hands turned beet red. His fingers stung when they thawed out inside the truck.

The storm paralyzed the city and brought residents to an abrupt halt. It was strange being the only ones out besides the city plows, front-end loaders, and the occasional cop car. The snow absorbed the road noise from our tires. It was like we were driving in a soundproof capsule through a tunnel. I couldn't see the sky, the sidewalks, or the curbs. Drifts covered road signs, hydrants, and parked cars. Everything was white.

The roads were treacherous. Gale force winds reached 79 miles per hour at Logan Airport. It wasn't far from where we were. Hanging traffic lights blew sideways, many were blacked out, and others were blinking yellow. Speedbumps weren't marked inside the housing development. They were invisible and when my father hit one, it blew the hydraulic line in the plow. Getting out of the truck to fix it came with its own set of hazards. Besides the driving visibility being only a couple of feet, he had to watch out for the ice-coated power lines that broke free of the poles. The live wires whipped in the air before being buried by the falling snow.

Fear Knocked — Jacqueline Sullivan Wyco

The storm was cited as one of the most severe blizzards in US history. We were in a state of emergency. Snow trapped 3500 cars, trucks, and tractor-trailers along Route 128. Exit ramps like ours, Great Plain Ave. near Channel 5 in Needham, and for miles beyond were blocked by vehicles who couldn't go any further. Drivers were stranded. Thousands lost power. My mother was home alone with my brother. We called her from on top of a snowbank on a payphone outside of a Dunkin Donuts. I talked to her after my dad. She said she had the wood stove going and had enough wood inside. They lost power, but she lit the kerosene lanterns, and we still had gas so she could cook on the stove.

My father and I were gone for about thirty-three hours straight. The blizzard of 1978 was a historic, and catastrophic storm. It took 100 lives. When we arrived home, my father called his parents. They lived a couple blocks over. They were managing. My father said he'd be over to plow and shovel them out soon. My father went to work the next day and was held overnight for overtime. My mother was on her own again. When the skies cleared, my mother dug a tunnel from the front stairs to the sidewalk. We had three flights of stairs. We were in the highest house on the street. But my mother had the endurance of an athlete. When we needed groceries, my mother got out my brother's sled. She bundled him up in his snowsuit and she and I dressed in layers and set out for Star Market. Feet of snow and drifts made one mile feel like three. My mother and I took turns pulling my brother when he got too tired to walk. He was only six years old. We passed neighbors pulling their sleds. The blizzard brought out kindness in people. Neighbors said hello and talked about the storm. It is a time that I will never forget. My mother and father truly embodied what it meant to be self-reliant.

My father spent his lifetime steering me, guiding me, and impressing upon me the skills to survive, and how to keep safe. These were the lessons that were a part of everyday life. The blizzard was one example.

We couldn't take a leisurely hike on a well-marked trail only two towns over in the Blue Hills without preparing an emergency kit and bringing a compass. But knowing how to read the compass wasn't enough. You needed a backup plan in case you were lost in the woods without one. He showed me how to find my direction by reading the sun. Look where the sun is before you go into the woods. How high it is in the sky can tell you the time. Where you stand in relation to it can show you the path to follow. If it was cloudy, look at the tree line. Take an odd-shaped boulder or hollowed-out tree, and use them as markers. Follow a stream if you're lost, and if you find you've walked in a circle, for heaven's sake, whatever you do, DON'T panic.

There was no such thing as a casual family lunch or dinner when we went out as a family. He liked to treat us when he was off. He loved Italian food, seafood, and ribs. But he wasn't fussy. He'd eat almost anything if he had to, but he loved a good thick steak. On special occasions, it was prime rib. It had to be quality and a portion that he could barely finish. He always sat facing the door, whether we were in an old brick building near Faneuil Hall, that he considered a fire trap, or at a new restaurant that just opened up. He was on constant alert, aware of his surroundings and then some. He scanned every building we entered. Within minutes, he knew every exit and had a plan in his head if ever a fire or emergency erupted. My mother was used to it and for me and my brother, it was normal.

My father instituted fire drills on weekends when he was home. We lived in the oldest house on the street, on top of a hill in a two-story wooden frame house that was already over 50 years old by the time I was 10. From my bedroom on the second floor, I could see the rooftops of our neighbors. I had three windows all in a row that looked over the front yard. Two sixty-foot Colorado blue spruces stood on each side of our front stairs. One stretched over the porch roof outside my bedroom. My room was at the peak at least 80 feet up from the street and my brother, a toddler at the time, slept in a room closer to my parents. With each fire drill, my father repeated the escape route first. The drill was repetitive, and always began the same way.

He said, "Ma will get John. You take care of yourself."

He said, "If there's a fire, don't go into the hallway. Stay in your room, don't open the door. Get down low and crawl to the window. Open it and climb out on the ledge. Wait there on the roof. You'll be safe until the fire department comes."

Then I had to get into my bed and wait until I heard the smoke detector alarm. That was my signal to go. I'd jump out of that bed and hit the floor, crawling on all fours with my face just hovering over the hardwood floor.

As fast as I could, I popped up below the window, opened it up, hoisted myself out onto the six-inch ledge of the roof, and waited for him to come in. He'd time me not just once, but multiple times in a row. Then he'd go through some pointers. He said, "Remember to stay low and if you're in a building and there's hardwood floor, feel for the lines and follow them. They'll lead you to a wall, window, or the exit."

That's how I learned everything. Through practice, through repetition.

⸻

Many lessons came from watching how my parents handled themselves under pressure. I remember my father telling my mother the names of the firefighters who got pink slips in their checks. His job was in jeopardy. He thought for sure, he'd be next. In "1981 the budget cuts of Proposition 2 ½, sent roughly six hundred and fifty police officers and five hundred and fifty firefighters home without a job."[5] "But a group laid off became arsonists hoping it would get the city to see that it needed to hire manpower back."[6] "There was little consideration among the group about the people who were getting hurt. It became an absolute game of cat and mouse. They were having fun. Members of the arson ring even cheered as they watched buildings burn."[7] From the Grunge, "The Untold Truth Behind The 1982 Boston Arson Spree."

My father was relieved when he learned he wouldn't lose his job. But for him and other firefighters who remained on the job, nothing could prepare them for what came next.

My father fought fires during the largest, most historic arson case in the country. The firefighters didn't have a chance to sit and eat supper or shut their eyes. On many night shifts, they ran from the time they arrived on their shift to the next morning. "The city was ablaze with nightly fires, sirens wailing through the streets, and people too afraid to sleep."[8] "It was the conspiracy of the nine men, including three Boston cops and a Boston firefighter, who burned Boston and surrounding communities in the early 1980s." From the book "Burn Boston Burn: The Largest Arson Case in the History of the Country."

"By using the information provided by Robert Groblewski, one of the arsonists, the Department of Justice indicted the seven other arsonists, leading to a range of prison sentences from 5 to 40 years imprisonment."[9] From Wikipedia, "The 1982 Boston Arson Spree."

Ladder 7 Meetinghouse Hill in Dorchester where my father was stationed was, at one point, the busiest firehouse in the nation. On nights when my father worked, my mother called him so my brother and I could say goodnight. She never gave us a reason to worry, even though she knew the danger. If he didn't answer, one of the guys yelled *Sully, outside phone.* The pay phone was next to the stairs that led up to the bunkroom. It was everyone's phone. The tones and taps echoed from the taproom around the corner. It was hard to hear him. In the background, every call across the city came in over the loudspeaker in the firehouse. We paid little attention to them until it was his turn to go out. Without fail, our conversation ended with the deep bellowing roar of the ladder truck and the trembling diesel engine. My father shouted over it, "We gotta run, I gotta go."

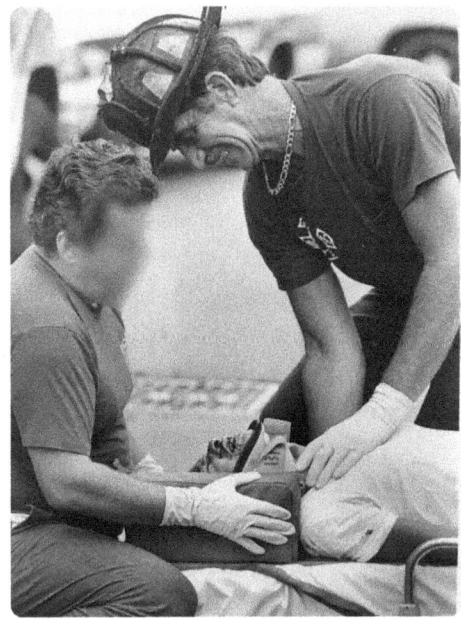

John (Sully, at right) grimaced as he's stabilizing the woman crying out in pain after a car crash.
From the Sullivan Family Photo Collection, photographer unknown.

If it was a working fire and early enough when he got back, he'd call us.

My father said, "Put the TV on channel five. Watch for me. I'm on the roof, opening it up."

Fires were always the top news story back then. We'd sit with our eyes glued to the portable RCA nine-inch black and white TV in the kitchen. Sure enough, we'd spot him on top of a three-decker opening up the roof, engulfed in smoke, with flames shooting out below. That's how we saw my father on many a night. He was larger than life, even on the tiny screen.

During my father's career, he fell through floors, got trapped on rooftops, and extracted people from horrific crashes. He pulled multiple people out of the fires. In those days, generations lived together in an apartment, and it wasn't uncommon to have five or six adults, more than one baby, and children of all ages, in one home fire. When my father came home safely, the next day after his night tour, he reeked of smoldering charred wood. It seeped out from his skin, hair, and his mustache. Over-exposure to smoke was normal for a firefighter. There were no oxygen tanks or masks when he started on the job. And after the safety gear was adopted, he saw them as more of a hindrance, as many firefighters did, in that era.

It didn't faze us when he got injured. My mother, brother, and I were happy when he was home. There was nothing in my mind that could take my father out. When he survived electrocution later in his career, in the early 1990s, he proved me right. He was lit up like a Christmas tree when pulling down a ceiling at a gas company fire. The power that was supposed to be shut off wasn't. The wire came down and wrapped around his head, chest, and arm as 220 volts raged through his body. And when a member of his crew grabbed my father's arm to free him, the force of electricity threw him several feet away. He got up, and he tried again. This time he charged my father like a linebacker, and he freed him. I found out while getting ready for work. I had the TV on in the background and when the news anchor said *John Sullivan,* I ran over to the screen. My father's arm hung off the stretcher. It swayed as they carried him to the ambulance. He was lifeless. But he survived unscathed. My father wasn't joking when he said he had nine lives. I believed him.

Over the years, sometimes a call bothered him, not because of the blood or gore as we often heard about, but the times when kids were involved, like my brother and me. A call on a bitter night was one of those times that stayed with my dad for years. Now and then he spoke of the little girl. Firefighters arrived at a house. The call came in as a kitchen fire. There was food cooking, but my father couldn't see it. Smoke filled the kitchen. The stovetop was covered. Piles of grease burned under crusted pans and caked-on filth. Trash bags were piled high to the ceiling, blocking the back door. The stench was awful. There were so many cockroaches. It looked as if the wall was moving.

Conditions like this weren't unusual, but this one was bad. When he looked around, he saw the little girl and his heart sank. He asked her where her room was. With her tiny hand, she took my father by one of his fingers and led him up the stairs to the attic. It wasn't just her room. Many used it for taking drugs and crashed there when they passed out. The dirty mattresses that covered the floor belonged in a dumpster, not for a kid to sleep on. There were no sheets or pillows, only a single blanket covered with stains.

He saw what most of us could never imagine. Neighborhoods seemed more like a war zone, where the innocent became the casualties on their streets and in their homes. My father felt for those who couldn't defend themselves, the ones who were powerless, victims of their condition. He tried but never found out what happened to the little girl. Now I wonder after all this time, did the little girl feel his heartbreak through her tiny little hand when he saw how she lived? And did she ever think of the firefighter later in her life, who she led up the stairs all those years ago?

Fear Knocked — Jacqueline Sullivan Wyco

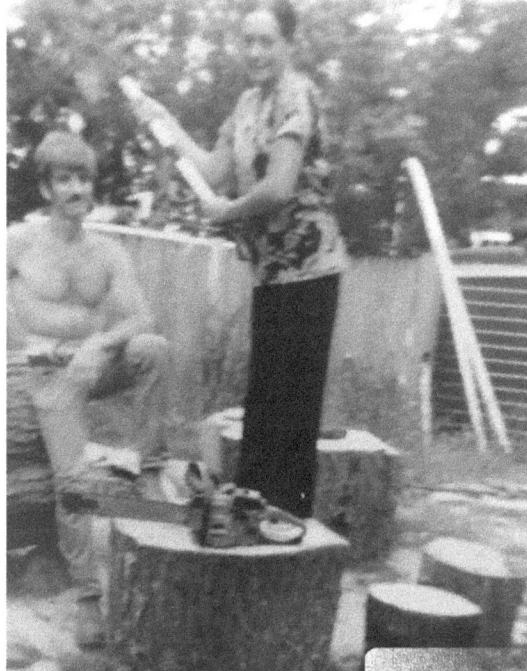

John (Sully) and Beverly(Sis) in the 1970s.
From the Sullivan Family Photo Collection

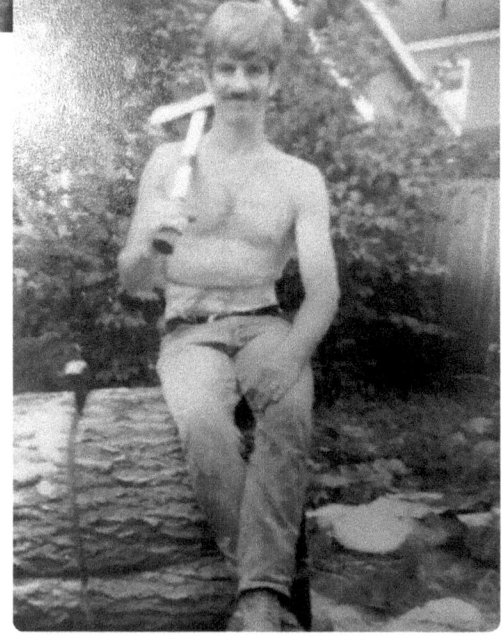

John (Sully) Sullivan 34 years old
From the Sullivan Family Photo Collection

Imprints From My Childhood

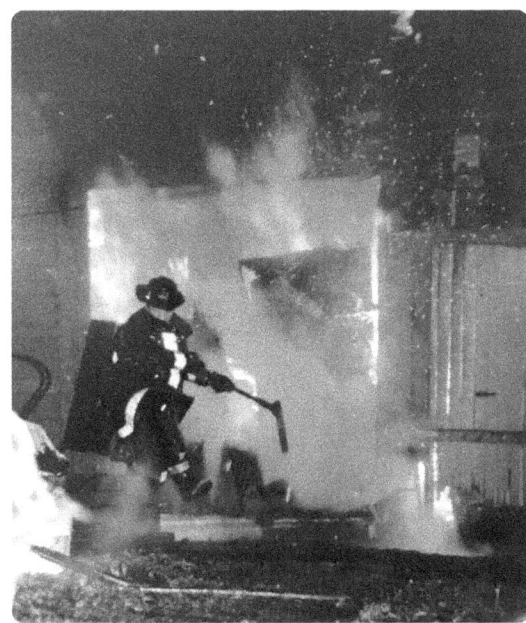

John (Sully) Sullivan using his favorite tool, the adze.
*From the Sullivan Family Photo Collection, **photographer unknown.***

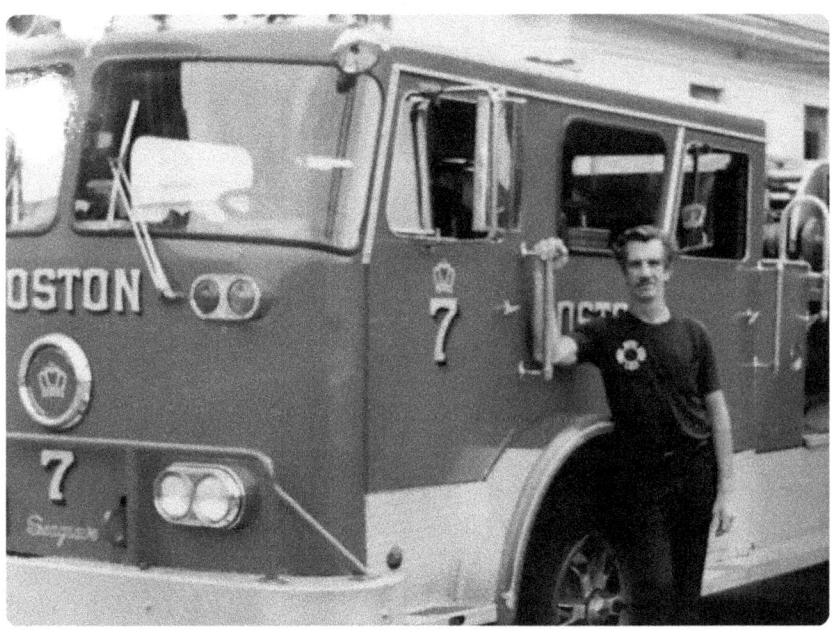

Ladder 7 Meetinghouse Hill Dorchester MA.
*From the Sullivan Family Photo Collection, **photographer unknown.***

Chapter 3
Love and Loss

Throughout my parents' marriage, their love grew stronger. My father came close to losing her once, and he didn't take her for granted. Often, he came home after work with flowers, just because. He usually worked side jobs in the mornings after his night tours. He finished concrete aprons on pools mainly in Revere, and Saugus. He'd go to lunch at Santarpio's in East Boston when he was over there. They made old-school Italian pizza pies. Then he'd make a special stop on the way home at the Modern Bakery in the North End for cannoli or my mother's favorite, lobster claw pastry if they weren't sold out. My father adored my mother and when I grew old enough to stay home alone with my brother, he took her away for a winter vacation, just the two of them. They went to Aruba, Cancun, Saint Martin, and Turks and Caicos before they became popular resort destinations. They were happy and after 32 years they were still very much in love.

At 49 years old, my mother's cancer returned. This time it was in her colon. My mother had surgery and recovered. Two years went by. She was cancer-free. She and my father were planning their future as he approached retirement age. Both were looking forward to traveling and spending more time together. In May of that year, my mother suddenly didn't feel right. She was the type of person who was up, dressed, and out the door, after my father left for work. She did her errands first thing in the morning, then occasionally, she was off to a few consignment stores that she loved to rummage through. But lately, she had no energy. Getting dressed was a chore, and nausea caused her to lose her appetite. She felt something was off. Her bloodwork

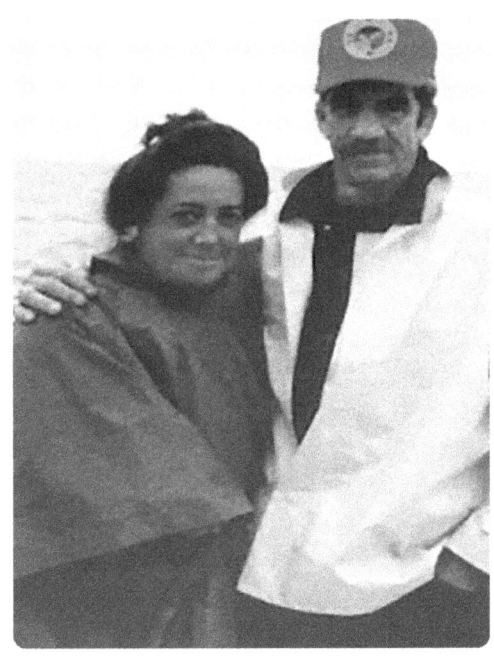

John (Sully) and Beverly (Sis) salmon fishing on Lake Ontario, New York in 1989
From the Sullivan Family Photo Collection

revealed diabetes. Nausea was treated as acid reflux, but the dull ache in her stomach soon traveled above her kidneys and lower back. Within a month, the pain turned stabbing. She tried to hide it. I remember watching her walk out of the kitchen into the hallway. She doubled over, took a deep breath, and came back into the room when the pain eased. I was worried. My mother went back to the doctor, but the tests performed didn't show cancer. Surgery was the only way to determine what was wrong.

In July 1992, my parents postponed their RV trip to the Blue Ridge Mountains in the Shenandoah Valley of Virginia. My mother's surgery revealed that cancer returned to her colon. Surgery removed it and she went home to recover. But she didn't get better. The pain intensified. My mother's favorite hobby was soaking in the sun from her lounge chair in our backyard. It rejuvenated her. She tried to sit out, but it made her too comfortable. I thought maybe scar tissue and adhesions were causing the pain. My mother asked me to take her for a ride. She thought a change of scenery might help her take her mind off the pain. I drove her along the rural Route 109, to Briggs Shady Oaks Dairy Farm in Medway. They bottled fresh milk there. My mother usually bought a gallon at a time for my brother, two quarts of white, and two quarts of chocolate. I pulled the car over near the farm under a big tree in the shade next to a stone wall. My mother reclined her seat all the way back. The grass in the field smelled sweet, like it was just mowed. She loved taking rides to places like this. And so did I. But this didn't make her feel better and the pain didn't subside. She was back in the hospital in early August for another surgery.

It poured sheets of rain the day my father, brother, and I waited in the hospital. About three hours in, we walked down to the cafeteria to pass some time. My father gazed into nowhere as he sipped his coffee. My brother and I did the same as we picked at our food. Two crows caught our attention when they flew down from a tree and stared at us in our booth. It was so eerie that the three of us got up and went back to the waiting area. The surgery lasted for more than seven hours, much longer than anticipated. We knew the news wasn't good when we saw the doctor's face. The cancer spread to my mother's liver and the part of her pancreas that she had left. When the doctors checked on her, she pulled out the respirator tube from her throat. She wanted to know the truth. When the doctor told her there was no chance of recovery, she asked that the tube be left out and the machines be turned off.

We stayed with her in the ICU, and I called her friends to say goodbye. She thanked them for their years of friendship. For one friend, she offered congratulations on her daughter's upcoming marriage, wishing them a good life. She said goodbye to each friend. They all had tears streaming down their cheeks when they opened the curtained-off partition. When they left, my father put a safety pin with a small medal of the Virgin Mary and one with Saint Michael on her pillow. My father, brother, and I told her it was okay for her to go. She opened her eyes and said, "I'm trying." Then the last rites were performed, and we waited. My father slept by her bed in a chair. My brother and I slept on top of a blanket on the floor. She hung on longer than expected. An incoming patient needed the bed in the ICU, so my mother was transferred to a private room. My cousin Jack came to visit us. He gave us special holy water that rolled under his car seat a couple of days before when his mother had given it to him to bring up for us. My aunt brought it home from her trip to the shrine in Medjugorje, Bosnia, years prior. My father opened the small bottle, put the water on his two fingers, and blessed my mother with the sign of the cross on her forehead. On the night of August 13, 1992, my mother, Beverly Sullivan, took one long breath, then another, and she was gone.

We knew it was inevitable, but we were in disbelief. My cousin went out into the hallway to get a nurse. Two came in and pronounced her time of death. We were escorted out of her room after a few minutes. We were still in shock when the nurse instructed us where to pick up the receipt to collect my mother's belongings. The elevator took us one floor down from the lobby to a caged office near the morgue. I don't know how to describe the feeling of picking up my mother's belongings.

The biggest part of our lives was gone. We handed over a receipt to get the tangible pieces of her that remained. A clear plastic bag filled with her clothing and a brown envelope with her jewelry were labeled with Beverly Sullivan written in black magic marker. The smell of her Shalimar perfume with the scents of sweet vanilla, jasmine, and sandalwood floated out from the top of the bag when I picked up the drawstring. I held it next to me and clutched the envelope as we walked to the truck in the parking lot. We were missing the person who was always there for us. Now we had to leave her behind. As we drove away, the full moon appeared as if it were moving. It lit the trees along the parkway and guided us like a headlight beaming from the sky. Then the moon stopped and hovered above our garage when we pulled into our driveway. It continued to guide us as it lit the path to the back door. When we walked into the house, my mother's death didn't seem real. She wasn't there and would never be again. At twenty-six years old, it felt like I had been catapulted back to the time my brother was born when my mother had to go back into the hospital. The separation gave me an overwhelming sensation of wandering alone. For my brother, at nineteen, my mother had been his best friend. My father went to sleep alone, and my brother and I laid blankets, and our sleeping bags on the floor, next to his bed. We couldn't bring ourselves to be apart.

I saw a part of my father's soul leave with her the night she died. My father's world had stopped. His spirit broke, and there he sat at the kitchen table for the first time in his life, unsure of what to do. My father was a widower at fifty-three years old. He was lost without my mother. He called me at work, multiple times a day, to check in. Most of the time, he'd be sobbing uncontrollably on the other end. This went on for months. I didn't know what to say. It was beyond awful, and I didn't know how he'd manage or if he could overcome it. His retired partner, Murray, helped my father immensely. He recommended a psychologist from the department to help him. Eventually, my father worked through his loss and went on living the best way he could without my mother, his best friend and soulmate. The pain and sorrow never fully healed and when he spoke of her, his deep brown eyes filled up with the love of the rarest kind.

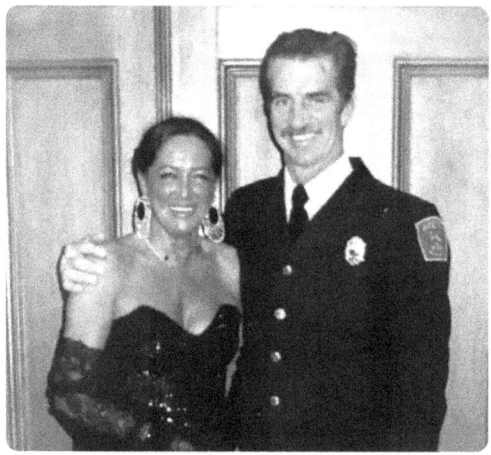

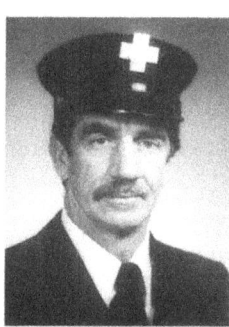

ROLL OF MERIT
is hereby awarded to

Fire Fighter John J. Sullivan
Ladder Company 7

Above, John (Sully) and Beverly (Sis) at a Boston Fire Department commendation ceremony recognizing John for a rescue in which he received the Roll of Merit (at right).

Photo from the Sullivan Family Photo Collection.

Roll of Merit, *Printed with verbal permission from the Boston Fire Department. Boston Fire Historical Society, Official Website*

On August 13, 1989, at 2110 hours, Ladder Company 7 responded to a building fire at 46 Lyons Street, District 7. Upon arrival fire was showing from the rear of a three story duplex on the second and third floors. Citizens informed Fire Fighters John J. Sullivan and John L. McKay, Jr., of Ladder Company 7, that a woman and her child were still in the second floor and a man, who had entered the building to search for them, had not returned.

Both fire fighters entered the building by the front door and made their way to the second floor via the front stairs. Upon reaching the second floor, Fire Fighter John J. Sullivan entered the left side apartment and conducted a room to room search through increasingly intense heat. He located a woman at the rear of the apartment who, in an extremely confused and nearly unconscious state, was holding an infant wrapped in a blanket. Fire Fighter Sullivan immediately removed them to safety, through the front of the building, to the street.

Simultaneously, Fire Fighter John L. McKay, Jr., entered the right side apartment of the second floor and conducted a room to room search through heavy smoke and intense heat. He located a man at the rear of the apartment, who was at floor level attempting to open the door to the rear stairway which was fully involved in fire. Fire Fighter McKay forcibly restrained the man from opening this door and removed him to the street through the front of the building.

Both of these rescues were performed before ventilation had occurred or lines were in place. Adding to the difficulty and confusion was the fact that the occupants were unable to speak English, making communication extremely difficult.

Because these rescues were performed at great personal risk, reflecting great credit upon themselves and the Boston Fire Department, the Fire Commissioner highly commended Fire Fighter John J. Sullivan and Fire Fighter John L. McKay, Jr., Ladder Company 7 in General Order No. 54 of 1989.

The Fire Commissioner, upon recommendation of the Board of Merit, orders that the names of F.F. John L. McKay, Jr. and F.F. John J. Sullivan, both of Ladder Co. 7, be placed on the Roll of Merit of the Boston Fire Department.

Chapter 4
Transformation

My father wasn't the type to feel sorry for himself. In his unrelenting search to move through his pain, he came across an ad in the Boston Globe that caught his attention. The Pan-Mass Challenge took place on the first weekend in August. It was a 190-mile bike ride from Sturbridge to Provincetown, a fundraiser to fight cancer. It was the catalyst that brought him back and moved him forward. He took every ounce of his grief over my mother and poured himself into the cause. Once the spring thaw hit, my father ventured out to ride his bike. He preferred the rural roads. Especially, those with little traffic, so he could concentrate on riding, not dodging cars. Climbing a hill that seemed to go on forever cauterized his pain. He healed as he peddled through the

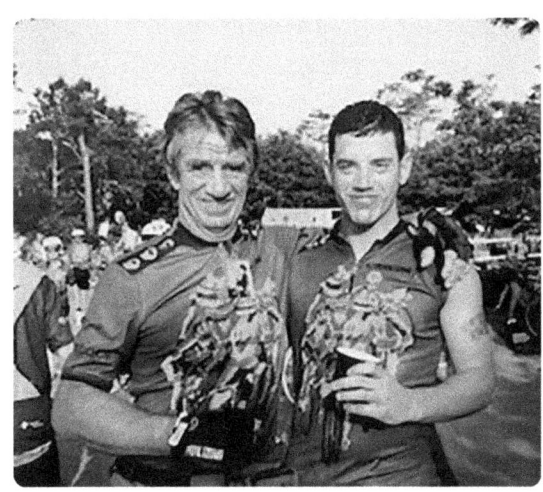

Author's father and brother John, Pan Mass Challenge 1995. See photo of the author's mother clipped to her father's shirt. (noted in this chapter)
Photo from the Sullivan Family Photo Collection

burning sensations in his legs and lower back. Most days, he trained alone. At first, he started slowly, about twenty-five miles, three times a week. Then gradually, throughout June and July, he'd work his way to fifty, seventy, and up to one hundred, which cyclists call a century.

My brother and I dropped him off on his first year riding in 1993, at the Sturbridge Host Hotel, the lodging and sign-in for riders. We didn't plan on it, but we stayed through the opening ceremonies. Every person who rode had a connection to the cancer cause. They were sons, daughters, nieces, nephews, friends, those in remission, and others who were cancer-free. All rode because of their connection and their commitment to finding a cure. Rows of tables filled the function room where dinner was served and for the speakers who followed. It was packed. My father, brother, and I found three open seats at a table near the back. My father introduced himself, and us to the riders we sat next to. Several guest speakers recounted their stories. I watched my father as the night progressed. The stories of each guest speaker brought tears to his eyes and ours. The opening ceremonies lifted and energized the spirit of what it means to come together for a cause. It transformed the grief we all shared into hope.

The next morning, before sunrise, a sea of almost two thousand cyclists transformed into a moving shrine. All adorned themselves with a memory, a picture, a name, or a row of names of those they rode for. My father had my mother's three-inch by two-inch picture laminated. He clipped it on the front left corner of his shirt, above his heart.

After that, my father rode every year without fail. So, when he told me he wanted to ride cross-country, I didn't doubt him. Once he decided, he never looked back. He was unwavering and relentless in any endeavor he tackled.

He remained in tremendous shape, and when he trained for this, he entered another level of fit. On the "Big Ride" Across America, he endured hazardous weather and unexpected dangers along the road. I gave him a diary and on page one he wrote:

> *Seattle to Easton 76.1 mi. June 15, 1998, Day 1*
>
> *About 10 miles into the ride a pallet came off a truck on the highway over our head and hit a rider*

right in front of me. He was all right but could have got killed. It was mostly mountain climbing. One mountain was 12.4 mi up at a six-degree grade and then the rains came. I got soaked and left my rain gear in my bag. A no-brainer. There was snow on top of the summit. It was breathtaking. As I was riding a trailer RV had a blowout and the tire flew all around me and I dodged two bullets in one day. Sleet and rain: had to bus 300 back to camp.

For six and half weeks, for 3,300 miles from Seattle, Washington to Washington, DC, the long and grueling ride paled compared to what my mother had gone through, my father said.

Day 11 in Montana. Physically demanding to say the least.

June 25th Missoula Mt to Avon 98.1 miles

It rained pretty heavy most of the morning as usual. I didn't have my pants or boot covers. It was 101 miles today. Pulled into a big gift store and coffee bar and dried out a little. Everyone was soaked. I started again slow so my legs wouldn't swell. I had two flat tires and didn't get to camp till 7 pm.

Day 12 in Montana took all the riders by surprise.

June 26 Avon to Townsend 62 mi

Today was the craziest yet. It started out dry. It rained a little last night but dry when we got up. Then the rain started. We left camp late, almost 6 am. We had to climb McDonald Pass. Altitude 6285 feet. The highest we would climb for the rest of the way. We started up about ½ way. I saw wet snow starting. Magan was behind me, and I told her jokingly about it. But the higher we climbed, the conditions got worse. Finally, when we got to the top it was like a whiteout and freezing cold. We had a pit stop on the top. We huddled together under two tents which gave us only relief from the fierce wind and cold. They said they were getting buses to take us down, so I took off on my bike six and a half miles down. What a ride. At times I had no brakes. It was the coldest ride of my life. I made it down only to be told we couldn't ride no more. I was bullshit. They took busloads of bikers to the hospital with hypothermia. It was really bad. Mike and George found a girl mumbling down at the bottom of the hill saying she had no brakes. She couldn't close her fingers. Her hands were pure white. They rushed her to a motel and got her warmed up and some pizza. Put her in a warm shower and when they went to pay for the room the manager wouldn't let them pay. These people are really great. Tomorrow, 4 of us are going back to where they sagged us and starting. Looks like a 130-mile day.

The next morning, he found a rancher and paid him to bring them back. He wanted to make sure he pedaled every inch of the way. My father was an unshakeable force.

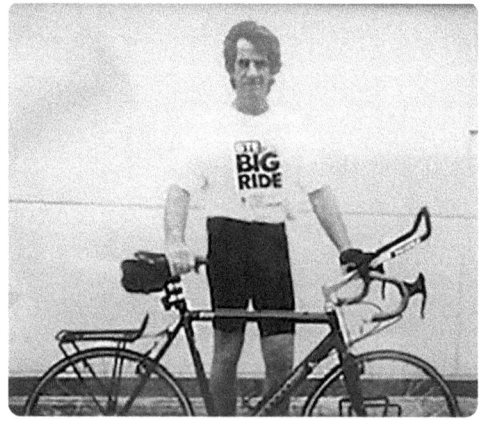

Day before leaving on the Big Ride, June 13, 1998.
From the Sullivan Family Photo Collection

Transformation

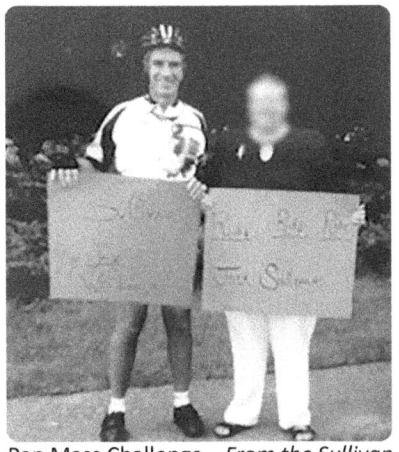

Pan Mass Challenge *From the Sullivan Family Photo Collection*

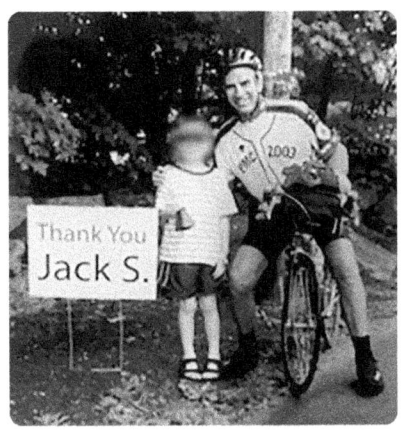

Pan Mass Challenge. After John's wife Beverly died, he was called Jack *From the Sullivan Family Photo Collection*

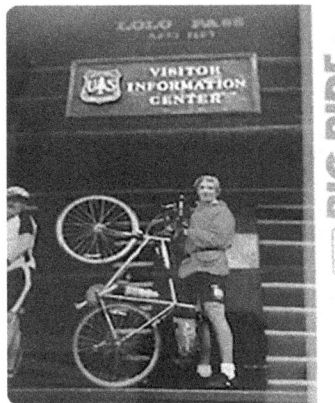

Big Ride in Montana June 1998
From the Sullivan Family Photo Collection

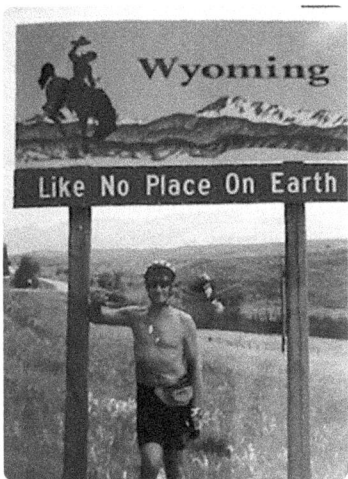

Entering Wyoming on day 17 of the Big Ride, July 1, 1998
From the Sullivan Family Photo Collection

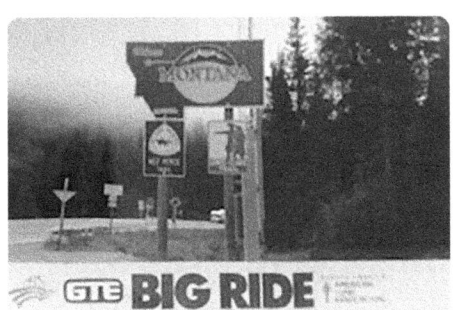

Entering Montana on day 9 of the Big Ride, June 23, 1998
From the Sullivan Family Photo Collection

Fear Knocked — Jacqueline Sullivan Wyco

My father introduced Marie to me at his house in 1998. She was three years older than my father, who was fifty-nine at the time. I saw from Marie's head to her manicured toes, she was conscientious of her appearance. Marie dressed in coordinating outfits. She put most of them together with odd pieces that complemented each other. She wore thick mascara and combed her white platinum hair, straight, below her ear. She joked and said it came from Loreal. She smiled like a model in a photo shoot, on demand, all teeth showing, and her eyes wide open when we met and every time after that.

My father loved music and dancing. When he decided it was time to date, he ventured out to the singles night at Mosely's on the Charles River. It was a famous ballroom right down the street from our house. It drew big bands and crowds from all over.

That's where he met Marie. She had been divorced for a few years and had two adult children. She worked at a Boston law firm and lived up on the North Shore. She had a variety of interests, such as art, the beach, and, of course, dancing. She preferred hotels over camping and walking in quaint villages over hiking on a nature trail. Marie hired a lady to clean her condo, rather than do it herself. And she preferred to eat out rather than cook. She appeared to be a regular working person with a full and busy life.

My father and she were going steady before he left on the Big Ride Across America. They seemed to hit it off. Mostly, they lived separate lives. My father had his home and his friends, and she had hers. My father spent most of his time cycling, fundraising, and traveling throughout Europe. Marie had a passion for art, wine, painting, shopping for clothes, and dining out. She became a regular presence in my father's life when he was home, and he enjoyed her company just as much as he enjoyed having his own space.

Marie shared a little of her past. Come to find out, I knew her son, as we both had worked in the same restaurant years prior. And I met her daughter and her husband at a party I invited them to after my father finished the Big Ride.

During the winters, my father was off to Florida, where he bought a small condo near West Palm Beach, on the Atlantic Coast, on the Intracoastal. Years of fighting fires and finishing concrete took their toll on his body and the sunny, warm weather was the cure for everything that ailed him. Marie kept in touch with him while he was there. She flew down periodically throughout the winter season.

Soon after my father returned in the spring, he and Marie visited my home on Cape Cod. She shared with me her love of the Cape.

She said, "I'd love to retire here. But I couldn't afford it on my own. It's beautiful here. So quaint and charming."

Over the years, Marie openly expressed her desire to live there. But she never spoke about making her dream a reality or if she intended to pursue it. And I never asked her.

Years passed before Marie divulged her plan. In 2009 we were at my father's celebrating his 70th birthday on a summer afternoon with family we hadn't seen in quite a while. All of us were catching up with each other and having a few laughs when the subject of bucket lists came up. Marie shared her dream of living on Cape Cod, but it was my first time hearing about how she would achieve this goal. She looked at my father.

She said, "If you sell this house and I sell mine, we could buy a place on the Cape."

At that instant, the mood shifted from light to uncomfortable. The conversation ended quicker than it began. My father was adamant he wouldn't leave his home. His irritation was palpable, and his reaction showed that he was familiar with her plan. My father was proud of his home. Boston was the city he loved. It's where he was born, raised his family and worked.

My father said, "My dead body will have to be carried out of here. I just finished the great room and a brand-new kitchen. I'm never leaving. I love it here."

My father finished renovating the kitchen. He opened up the entire space and installed granite countertops, maple cabinetry, and heavy-duty appliances. The kitchen flowed into the great room. It was everything he envisioned. Twelve-foot-high stained wood, natural ceiling with a panoramic arched picture window showcased his backyard of flowers and concrete red brick stamped driveway he had put in with help from his friends in the local. The four skylights were electric. They automatically closed if it rained. The triple sliding glass door led out onto a twenty-by-twenty deck with an eight-person Jacuzzi hot tub. His home was his castle. He wasn't leaving, selling, or going anywhere. And in his body language, and emphatic NO, he made it clear.

I don't remember what Marie said. All I remember was the model-like smile she made from ear to ear. My father's reaction took most of my focus off Marie. My father created his life, and he was content. Several times he mentioned he very much liked Marie but had no interest in selling his home or marriage and he was upfront with her about how he felt.

My father was disciplined throughout every area of his life, including his finances. Money symbolized hard work because that's how he earned it. When his bills arrived, he sent them out. My father didn't put them aside, nor did he wait and pay them closer to the due date. He didn't owe a cent, and he always thought before he spent. He knew how to save, and he lived within his means. In his eyes, money wasn't something he wished for, and he didn't begrudge other people for having it. But Marie didn't share all his views.

One night, years later, after I met my husband and married in 2010, my brother and I, with our spouses, got together at my father's house for dinner with Marie. During one conversation, Marie mentioned my father had "plenty of money." The mood shifted immediately. It almost seemed like a derogatory remark. I felt the bitterness swirl in the air when she said it. More than once this happened, and over the years, and in every instance, when she made this statement, I felt the same cringe. If this statement was fleeting, it would have meant nothing, but because it was repetitive, it revealed a deeper fixation Marie had. I always thought that it was just Marie being Marie. At first, it seemed like Marie had her quirks and faults like anyone else. But she minimized what my father valued. And in general, she often appeared to accept what she didn't want to hear, through a smile, but, then she'd make a subtle remark that bordered on joking and insulting. It was hard to tell. Was she kidding or was her habitual use of sarcasm and backhanded comments a deeply engrained behavioral pattern used to mask her true inner feelings?

As for my father, there was no mistaking what he felt. He wore all his emotions visibly. My father lived life with purpose. He set goals, and he planned his future. Without mincing his words, he always spoke from his heart. Yes, you could even say he was hard-headed, but one thing about my father was there was no point in trying to sway or persuade him. If he made a well-thought-out decision, he wouldn't budge. Especially when it involved a deep personal connection and/or belief that he had.

My father accepted Marie as she was. Besides, his relationship was just that, his. Ultimately, he had the power to choose who he wanted to be in his life. He could take care of himself. After all, I knew my father. He had a boundary. He called it quits with girlfriends before he dated Marie. He could read a face, a handshake, and in a few words, he knew if a person was genuine.

My father had a keen sense and a healthy dose of self-esteem. He respected himself and didn't allow others to take advantage of him. But unbeknownst to my father, that was all about to change. His once acute judgment was about to grow impaired. Alzheimer's was on his doorstep and soon, all his boundaries would disintegrate. And there would be no escape from what was happening inside of his brain.

LESSON LEARNED

"Alzheimer's disease begins long before any symptoms become apparent. This stage is called preclinical Alzheimer's disease. This stage of Alzheimer's can last for years, possibly even decades. Although you won't notice any changes, new imaging technologies of the brain can identify amyloid plaques and neurofibrillary tangles. The tangles develop when tau proteins change shape and organize into structures. These are hallmarks of Alzheimer's disease."[10] From the Mayo Clinic, "Alzheimer's Stages: How the Disease Progresses."

Chapter 5
Alzheimer's, The Warning Signs

The year 2003 marked five years since the Big Ride. Life for a while seemed to flow on an even keel, and it was nice. My father and Marie were still dating. He was busy cycling and traveling through Germany. He flew to California, to see his friends from the Big Ride. They traveled together throughout the years to Europe, and out west in the US. They had a mutual interest in the places where Native Americans, soldiers, and ordinary people made history.

My father called me to check in two or three times a week. I told him about a job offer that opened at a large rehab facility down the street from him. He offered to let me stay at the house during the week. Rush hour traffic turned a one-hour commute into two, to my home on the Cape.

He said, "Your room is always there for you. Whenever you want to stay."

And after a few weeks of battling bumper-to-bumper traffic, I

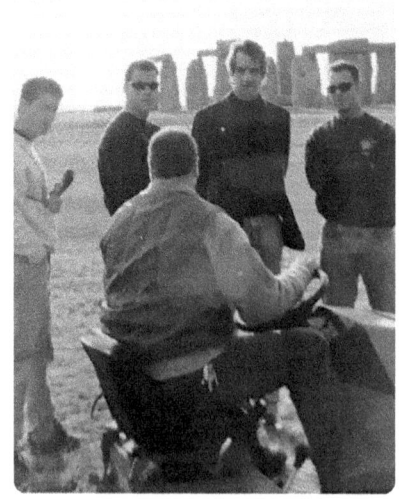

Stonehenge, Wiltshire England
From left to right John's friends from California Joe Novelli, Mike Keefe, John (Jack) Sullivan, Dave Cowan.
Photo from the Sullivan Family Photo Collection.

took him up on it. Home was comforting, and in retrospect, life gifted me the opportunity to live with him again.

From 2003 to 2008, I witnessed in my father the initial stages of Alzheimer's disease, an illness I never expected. Even though I was living with him, I didn't have a clue his symptoms were not the signs of what I thought to be normal aging. At sixty-four years old, he was ten years away from his formal diagnosis. The communication signals in his brain had already faltered. He didn't look sick. He had the blood pressure of a twenty-year-old, and he was the picture of health.

However, the decline in his cognitive function had already crept to the surface, and it affected every aspect of his life. Alzheimer's went undiscovered. In reality, my father suffered from a slow-moving, unrelenting, and merciless disease. A storm of uncertainty raged, and eventually, it would wipe out the rock-solid stability that ran through his veins.

My father had a problem remembering, so he did what he always did. He came up with a solution. He started with yellow sticky notes. Then he added an extra-large desk-sized calendar. He always had a backup to a backup. This backup reminder he put in his car. It was a suction-cupped device that stuck to the windshield. It came with a pen attached and a pad that he placed right in the middle of the dash. It didn't matter how many reminders, or how many notes he posted around, he still missed appointments. Mishaps like this kept happening. One day, my father rubbed his head and said out loud, "I don't know what's wrong with my head."

He felt like he was in a fog. And he couldn't get out of it. His brain was changing. Out of the blue, it seemed, he began suffering from migraines. Some were so debilitating they knocked him out for two or three days.

Forgetting caused frustration. When we were out, he routinely bumped into someone he knew. I noticed over time his recall was growing worse, especially with people's names. It bothered him when he forgot them. He felt embarrassed and tried to work around the conversation so the person wouldn't notice. I saw how he beat himself up. He felt ashamed. When we got into his car, he hit the steering wheel with his hand as he forced himself to remember. But forcing it pushed it further away. He just couldn't get it to come out. He racked his brain as we drove away until it came to him, but it was always too late.

He said, "Why couldn't I get his name when I was talking to him? I had it. I just couldn't get it to come out."

There was a place for everything and everything in its place, but that too, fell to the wayside for my father. Misplacing things, especially car keys, became more common. One morning after he and Marie stayed at my house, he couldn't find his keys. They were packed and ready to leave, but his keys were nowhere to be found. He had to take my truck, drive an hour back home to get his spare key, and come back. Only to find them in the fridge on top of a to-go container. He put them there as a reminder not to forget his food. I heard the anxiety in his voice, and I saw it on his face. He was hard on himself because he thought he should have been able to remember even when Alzheimer's was to blame.

Then there was the tipping point when he had trouble sleeping. He went to his primary care physician, and she prescribed him sleeping pills. One didn't work, so he took another, then another. I don't know if it was an alignment of events that collided, but after taking Ambien, my father attempted suicide. I don't know how or why this happened, but I do know that the warning label stated that Ambien could cause suicidal thoughts and actions. "Studies have shown that sleep deprivation and insomnia are associated with the pathogenesis of Alzheimer's disease and may have an impact on the symptoms and development." From the National Library of Medicine case study, published on March 17, 2022, "Sleep and Alzheimer's: The Link."[11] His physician didn't make the correlation between insomnia and Alzheimer's. Neither did any other physician. And the link between Ambien and suicidal thoughts and actions was overlooked. I firmly believe there was a connection. My father never had a history of suicide attempts. But there were definite changes in his brain and the facts led to Alzheimer's.

On the Friday afternoon before Thanksgiving 2005, I came in from work, and my father seemed unusually quiet. He sat on the couch and stared at the TV, but it wasn't on. As soon as I saw him, I felt something off with him.

I said, "What's wrong?"

Alzheimer's, The Warning Signs

He said, "Nothing, I'm fine. I just came in from putting wreaths up on all the graves for Christmas. I went to Ma's, my parents, my sister and Granny's."

He wasn't himself, and I didn't know if I should go home, but he insisted he was okay.

I said, "If you need anything, call me."

And I headed home for the weekend. I left an old family photo album sitting next to the couch on a chest at my father's. I had taken it down from inside the little room behind the fridge to make a collage and I didn't put it away. My father hadn't looked at pictures in the albums since my mother died. Before I understood Alzheimer's symptoms could appear decades before diagnosis, I thought my father's suicide attempt was triggered by the photos and putting Christmas wreaths on all our family graves.

My father had been on my mind all weekend. I had spent two days Christmas shopping, and unexpectedly I came across a concrete fire hydrant. Two men noticed it as I put it on my cart. They were intrigued and asked who it was for. I talked about my father that day to strangers. I believe on some level there was a message being sent my way.

It was Sunday night, about 5:30. I had just driven over the Sagamore Bridge on my way back to the house. I called my father to see if he wanted me to pick up supper. When he answered the phone, his voice sounded labored.

He said, "I need you."

I said, "What's going on?"

"I'm going to kill myself. I've got the shotgun in my hand."

My mind braced itself and fear shot through me like a jolt of lightning.

I said, "You can't do this."

This wasn't a problem I could think through, and I did not know how to get my father out of this. I couldn't rip the gun out of his hands while driving my truck on the highway, an hour away. I reacted.

I said, "If you do, you can forget about seeing Ma. She will never forgive you for this. Are you sitting down?"

He said, "No."

"Go in the kitchen, sit down in your chair, put the gun down and don't you dare move. I'm calling the police and when I call you back, you better pick up that phone."

My mother meant everything to my father, and in an instant, she became the solution, the power who could convince him to stop. Driving as fast as I could, I called the police, and I told them what was happening. I told Dispatch I had to call him back and that I would stay on the line with him until they got there. I called my father. He answered.

"The police are on their way and I'm going to stay on the phone with you until they get there."

When he grew quiet, I asked him what he was doing. It sounded like he got up from the chair. I asked him if he was pacing, and when he said yes, I told him to sit back down. There was an incoming call, and I told my father I'd be right back. It was the police. They were there. I got back on the line with my father.

I said, "They're outside. Dad, let them in."

They took him to Faulkner Hospital where I met him. I arrived to find him in a curtained-off section of the emergency room in a white straitjacket. He trembled and shook uncontrollably.

My father said, "I don't know if I'm getting out of this one."

For the first time in my life, I didn't know either. I stood beside him, in disbelief and put my hand on his shoulder. My father had this uncanny ability to pull himself out of every situation, but this felt like quicksand.

I called my brother, and he came up to the hospital right away. He hadn't been home at my father's, for the weekend either. He was just as shocked as I was. While at the hospital, I called Murray, my father's friend, and partner in the fire department. He was a great help to my father and my family after my mother died and he kept anything I shared with him in the strictest of confidence. Murray made a few calls and got him into McLean Hospital, the best hospital for what my father needed. There, he went through the beginning stages of recovery as an inpatient. Murray visited regularly and so did my brother and me.

Marie had flown out of Boston the previous week. She went to visit a relative. I called to tell her what happened when I got home from the hospital. As I told her, there was complete silence.

I said, "Marie, are you still there?"

I thought the call had dropped. She listened but didn't ask how or why it happened. Our exchange was strange and brief, and I just told her I wanted to let her know what happened and that my father was safe in the hospital being monitored.

I don't know what was going through her mind or what her conversation with my father entailed before she left. But I got the feeling that something wasn't quite right between them. Marie's silence felt strange to me. Her decision to keep her distance around this time and during my father's recovery pointed to the fact that their relationship was at some sort of impasse. What I suspected was confirmed while she was still away. My father brought up their relationship when I visited him. He told me he was thinking of breaking it off with her. I asked him why and he said he didn't know. He gave no reason, and I didn't pressure him to tell me. I can't say what happened between them, I can only speculate. And I won't do it here.

The doctors at McLean Hospital diagnosed my father with anxiety and depression, and for months, he endured the medication roller coaster. The initial meds put him in what I can only describe as a lucid coma. He came home after a couple of weeks, and he continued to go to McLean for counseling and medication adjustments on an outpatient basis. He experienced an upswing.

However, just when he would start feeling good and level out, his signs of agitation would rise again, leading to further adjustments in his meds. Some medications caused extreme fatigue, so much so, it took everything he had to get out of bed, something he never had experienced before. I came home one day after work to find him lying on the couch. He hadn't been out all day.

I said, "Why don't you go for a walk? You need to get up and out. Exercise will make you feel better."

He said, "I don't feel like it."

I said, "Dad, just walk to the end of the driveway and back."

He said, "No. I don't want to."

It was frustrating for both of us. I wanted my father back. The will of a man is a powerful thing, and I knew he had it in him. What I didn't know was that his brain had most likely already begun changing on the cellular level. When I pushed him, it caused friction between us. I hated being at odds with him. The next day, my father came to visit me at work. We both felt bad for getting upset with one another.

"I'm sorry, Dad."

"I'm sorry, too, Jacqueline. I'll try harder."

We hugged, and both said, *I love you.*

My father knew what recovery entailed, and the steps he needed to take. He had done AA and stayed sober for over three decades. However, he struggled hard to move forward from this. It seemed almost too great to overcome. There was a laundry list of possible side effects from the meds he took. These medications, although necessary, made him feel groggy and spacey. So, he stopped taking them to feel better. He was in Florida at the time, with Marie, when he became more restless, agitated, and on edge. Marie decided she wanted to leave Florida, and they both came home earlier than usual. When they arrived at my father's, she dropped him off and left. I was surprised to see Marie's car gone when I pulled up the driveway after work. I walked into the kitchen and saw my father at the kitchen table.

I said, "Dad, what are you doing at home? What happened?"

He said, "My head was swimming, and I couldn't stand it, so I stopped taking the medication."

I said, "You just can't do that. You can't stop cold turkey, Dad. There are serious side effects. You have to take your pills."

He took them over to the kitchen sink, where he got a glass of water and when he walked away, I went over and put my hand down the garbage disposal and pulled up his pills. I called Murray two seconds later.

He had to go into McLean, but it wasn't as easy as making a phone call. There was a wait to get in. Murray made a call, and we got an appointment to see a physician. In our meeting, I expressed the need for my father to be readmitted and I also knew there was a chance they may not take him. Thankfully, they did.

My father never gave up, and he did the hard work of recovery. He got better, but I question his sleeplessness, anxiety, and depression. I wonder if these were the precursor symptoms to Alzheimer's and if it was his brain, somehow crying out for help way back then. I am convinced it was.

It took a solid year for my father to regain his footing and life resumed at a new normal. My father stayed with Marie, and they were spending more time together. He was active again, biking and dancing again, but it seemed my father grew accident-prone. His balance was off. He became increasingly unsteady, and this carried over to just walking. I noticed his tendency to trip over the slightest uneven section of sidewalk or irregular paved surface.

"Broadly defined, visuospatial function refers to the ability to identify, integrate, and analyze space and visual form, details, structure, and spatial relations in several (usually two or three) dimensions."[12] "In addition to core memory deficits, visual impairments are also pervasive in Alzheimer's."[13] "Based on the evidence accumulated to date, Alzheimer's is now recognized as a continuous process that begins 15 to 20 years before clinical symptoms emerge."[14] From the National Library of Medicine case study on February 9, 2021, "Stereoscopic Depth Perception and Visuospatial Dysfunction in Alzheimer's Disease."

Every symptom within my father's body signaled something much more serious. However, the signs were diagnosed as individual symptoms and treated individually, not holistically. His body was communicating with him. He felt something was off, but he too, didn't understand what was happening. When I look at the warning signs for Alzheimer's, the time frame before his diagnosis, and my father's symptoms, the answer screams off the page.

LESSONS LEARNED

When multiple signs begin appearing more regularly it's time for an evaluation.

"Early symptoms of Alzheimer's dementia include:
- Memory impairment, such as trouble remembering events.
- Having a hard time concentrating, planning, or problem-solving.
- Trouble finishing daily tasks at home or work, such as writing or using eating utensils.
- Confusion with location or passage of time.

- Having visual or spatial issues, such as not understanding distance in driving, getting lost, or misplacing items.
- Trouble with language, such as not being able to find the right word or having a reduced vocabulary in speech or writing.
- Using poor judgment in decisions.
- Withdrawal from work events or social engagements.
- Changes in mood, such as depression or other behavior and personality changes.

When warning signs of Alzheimer's dementia appear, it's important that you get a prompt and accurate diagnosis."[15] From the Mayo Clinic, "Diagnosing Alzheimer's: How Alzheimer's Is Diagnosed."

Chapter 6
The Progression

As new studies surface and science dissects Alzheimer's, I'm now able to see my father's decline unfold in the decade leading up to his diagnosis.

My father's immune system grew weaker and at sixty-three years old, fighting off the common cold wasn't as easy. Out of nowhere it seemed, he developed allergies. His sinuses grew chronically congested and inflamed. They were so bothersome that he went to a specialist at Mass Eye and Ear Hospital, where they discovered polyps and a deviated septum. The operation gave him some relief, but sinus infections happened more frequently. Augmentin, Flonase, and saline washes worked short term, but many times the sinus infection turned into bronchitis. Prednisone tapers and Z packs became part of a prescribed cycle that continued for the rest of his life. My father's chronic sinus condition could have been a contributing factor to his Alzheimer's.

My father's allergies spiked around the age of sixty-five: they were so severe that his doctor recommended he try immunotherapy. He periodically lost his sense of smell and one day, it vanished completely.

Researchers at the University of Chicago found a possible link between a gene associated with Alzheimer's disease and losing the sense of smell at around the age of sixty-five. The researchers think losing your sense of smell around that age could be an early warning sign of neurodegenerative disease.[16] From Verywell Health online magazine, "Losing Your Sense of Smell May Be a Warning Sign of Alzheimer's."

However, Alzheimer's doesn't cause the loss of smell. "In this case-control study of 22 patients with chronic rhinosinusitis and 22 healthy controls, participants with sinonasal inflammation showed decreased brain connectivity within the frontoparietal network, a major functional hub."[17] From the Journal of American Medical Association, "Association of Sinonasal Inflammation with Functional Brain Connectivity."

A rash that wouldn't go away developed on my father's face. They added a diagnosis of rosacea to his growing list of conditions for which he had no family medical history. It came as a surprise to me when I found research that linked rosacea and Alzheimer's. "Accumulating studies showed that rosacea develops as a manifestation of systemic illnesses that are linked to metabolic, psychiatric, and neurologic disorders, including Alzheimer's disease."[18] From the National Library of Medicine, "Bioinformatics and Network Pharmacology Identify the Therapeutic Role and Potential Mechanism of Melatonin in AD and Rosacea."

In 2007, after thirty years of cooking, I felt burned out. I needed and wanted a change from the constant mental and physical demands of being a hands-on chef. A polarity therapist came to give the residents where I worked a talk about her practice. I stopped for a few minutes to listen after I had served lunch. Energy work, massage therapy, and holistic healing always interested me and that night when I went home, I researched schools. Within a couple of weeks, I enrolled in night classes. Fourteen months later I was a licensed massage therapist.

In 2008, I resigned from my chef position and moved back to my home on Cape Cod full-time. I looked forward to starting my business. I went from seeing my father five days a week to only once every couple of weeks.

We spoke often, and most of the time we called just to say hi. If I called him before noon, his phone went automatically to voicemail. His morning ritual of getting up early, running errands, and grabbing a coffee at Dunks had taken on a new order that now began in the early afternoon. He attributed this new habit to years of sleep deprivation from working two jobs.

My father's prescribed nighttime med along with the medication for anxiety and depression could be one explanation for the changes in his sleep pattern. But before the suicide attempt and the diagnosis of anxiety, and depression his primary care physician prescribed Ambien. I don't know how long he had trouble sleeping, but I do know that my father wouldn't have sought out medication if this only happened occasionally.

I'm not sure why my father had trouble sleeping. He wasn't tested to see if it was a disorder and there is research that shows the connection between sleep disorders and Alzheimer's. "Sleep disorders are common in patients with Alzheimer's disease and can even occur in patients with amnestic mild cognitive impairment, which appears before Alzheimer's disease. Sleep disorders further impair cognitive function and accelerate the accumulation of amyloid-B and tau in patients with Alzheimer's disease. At present, sleep disorders are considered as a risk factor for, and maybe a predictor of, Alzheimer's disease development." [19] From the National Library of Medicine, "Sleep Disorders in Alzheimer's Disease: the predictive roles and potential mechanisms."

There were days my father sounded off when we talked. He seemed unengaged and distant. And I worried about him when he didn't seem like himself. The fact is Alzheimer's had already begun to disconnect my father from his world.

My father came to visit me at the Cape with Marie at least two or three times during the summer. Marie had grown out her hair and began wearing it as my mother used to, in a classic updated Victorian-styled bun. Marie loved the Cape, and she enjoyed coming to my house. I enjoyed being with them. When they came, Marie always brought her wine and enjoyed a glass or two while my father had his coffee, tea, root beer, or Coke.

They always stayed over for the weekend in between the other weekends that Marie had booked. She made the itinerary and that was fine with my father. When they were at my house, we'd go out for dinner, to the beach, or take in some local events happening around the Cape that Marie planned. Marie always seemed agreeable. But again, my father rarely disagreed with her about where to go, and it didn't make a difference to me. The visit was about being together, not about what we did.

No matter where Marie went, including the beach, she had her makeup on and wore all her favorite gold and silver jewelry. One Saturday, Marie suggested we go to the beach. Marie worked hard to maintain her figure. Marie, in her sixties, was in better shape than a lot of women her age and younger. She wore a two-piece bikini and made herself up in the usual fashion.

I suggested Old Silver Beach in Falmouth. It wasn't too far, and we packed up my truck and drove there for the afternoon. After we set up our chairs, I noticed my father seemed restless. He tapped his large gold ring on the arm of the chair, and he adjusted the back, up and down every few minutes. The beach had always been his place to unwind. In the past, within minutes he'd settle in on the sand. He soaked up every ray as if he had never seen the sun, every single time he went. He loved it that much. But this time, he couldn't relax.

When my father went to the bathroom, I asked Marie how she thought he was doing. Had she seen and felt what I just did? She saw it too, but didn't go into any detail. When my father came back, I asked him, "Dad, do you want to go for a walk?"

"Are you okay, Dad? You seem a little anxious."

He said little and skirted around the conversation.

He said, "Yeah, I'm fine."

But he wasn't fine, and I suggested he call the doctor and follow up.

I said, "Dad, maybe you just need a medication adjustment. You don't have to feel like this. You may have leveled off. The meds can help you feel better."

But the meds couldn't help because they were treating a symptom of a diagnosis that no one could see. When my father wasn't doing well, I worried. When he felt good, like his old self, I felt better.

In 2009, I met my future husband Mark through a friend. Riley had been visiting her girlfriend for the weekend on the Cape. We were both at the same party and she and her friend were discussing their boyfriends on the Worcester Fire. I added my father had been on the Boston Fire. The small talk ran its course and then she questioned my relationship status, which at the time was single.

It was a while since my last relationship, and I decided it was time I started dating again. Riley told me she knew this great guy. I thought to myself. *Yeah, if he's so great, why is he single*?

Riley didn't wait. She texted him as we talked and asked him to send a picture. Then she snapped one of me and sent it to him. I looked at him and said to myself, *oh, he looks a little old.*

He told me later that when he looked at my picture, he thought, *what the heck, I'll take a ride to the Cape.*

When he called me from work, the sounds were all so familiar. The tones echoed in the background, and when I heard Ladder 7, I asked him if that was his truck. What were the chances? When I told him later that my father retired from Ladder 7, he couldn't believe it either. After we talked for a week or so, he asked if I wanted to get together. He wanted to drive to the Cape. After I said okay, I kind of panicked.

"Bring your fishing rod, in case you get bored. I can sit in my lounge chair and read a book or something down at the canal while you fish."

I wanted an option that didn't involve the pressure of conversation. Before Mark arrived, I took Kodi, one of my two German Shepherds out for a walk down to Peter's Pond. I thought he was further away when he texted. I saw his truck in my driveway as I crossed the road. He knocked a few times and thought I didn't answer the door on purpose. When he turned to go back to his truck, he saw me and walked towards me over the front lawn. I invited him in and we sat in my kitchen making small talk. As I listened to him, I felt comfortable and at ease.

It was Palm Sunday, a week before Easter. It rained the night before and I could see the sun coming out through clouds blowing out towards the sea from my skylight. It was turning out to be the perfect Spring day. I asked him if he wanted to take a ride to Scusset Beach, a state park down on the canal, just over Sagamore Bridge. My father took us camping in our trailer there when we were kids. Back then, we fished off the jetty, played softball on the beach, and rode our bikes along the canal as boats drifted through. Ever since, it has been my favorite place. I parked on the jetty side, next to the canal, and we walked along the beach, then sat on my tailgate and had a beer. I asked about his past and what he wanted for the future.

Mark went to school in upstate New York at Paul Smith's College, where he majored in forestry and park management. He wanted to be a park ranger. We had very similar interests. I had applied off Cape for a full-time park ranger position, but the pay wasn't enough to live on. Each of us had the dream of building a home on a piece of land in the woods. I had a catalog of cabin kits, and he had a book on how to build one.

He logged out in Colorado and lived in a tent for four months, then the company moved, so he ended up back home where he got a job with Bartlett Tree Company. They wanted to promote him as manager, but for the money they offered him, he quit and started his own tree business.

I pelted him with questions. *How long were you married? Why did your marriage break up?*

He expected a casual conversation, nothing intense. I told him I wanted to find out the kind of person he was, and I didn't want to waste time figuring him out. During our ten-hour date, we laughed, ate, and drove around in his truck, seeing some sights. He ended up calling in sick to his night shift, something he never did. When he pulled out of my driveway, I missed him. Mark had just become a part of my life.

About six weeks after dating, I asked my father if he wanted to meet him. I had told Mark all about him. At forty-four, I felt more like a teenager bringing home a new boyfriend than an adult. I was nervous, but Mark and my father had more than enough in common. During dinner, my father asked Mark about his life and how he got on the job. Just like my father, he hadn't planned on becoming a firefighter.

I never grew tired of listening to the stories my father told. He had to stop a few times when he mixed up the order of the details.

When he corrected himself and got back on track, I read nothing into it. Stories about fires. That could take hours to talk about, and still, there would be more stories to tell.

Then the mood became more somber when my father asked Mark how many children he had. Mark's twenty-month-old daughter died from a brain tumor. Mark explained that he healed through his loss by getting involved in the support group that had helped him. Within minutes, my father looked at me and he saw the type of guy Mark was. He was steady and strong, and he had values. A few months later, Mark asked for my father's blessing before we got engaged. He showed deep respect and valued my father's approval. It was an old-fashioned gesture that my father appreciated. I wanted to include Marie in my wedding and asked her if she would walk me down the aisle with my father. I considered her family, and I thought she felt the same way.

After our wedding, both Mark and I decided to forgo a honeymoon. We came home after our weekend wedding, and I started my new business, and he studied to be a lieutenant. I lived in Worcester, a city I knew nothing about. Getting used to it, and my new family took all my attention and my focus drifted away from my father.

It wasn't until 2015 that I learned of my father's Alzheimer's, and in the three years leading up to my discovery of his disease, I did not see my father as often. I was building a new business and just moved into a new home. When I saw him, I noticed a decline in his memory. I thought it was normal. Marie was always there by his side. She transitioned his pauses by finishing his thoughts. In the late fall of 2015, Marie revealed to Mark and me that she sat with my father in the doctor's office when he got the results. They didn't inform my brother and me about his diagnosis. My father saw Alzheimer's as something he could handle himself with Marie. But in doing so, he made himself more vulnerable than he already was.

The risks associated with this disease are terrifyingly real. Just Google, *financial abuse, and exploitation of people with Alzheimer's*, and a multitude of articles will bombard the screen. No one with

Alzheimer's is immune from such threats. Crimes against the cognitively impaired are rampant and surging out of control in the US and elsewhere. It's an epidemic, and, in my mind, these crimes have become as much a significant part of the disease as the physical symptoms themselves.

By not creating financial safeguards at the onset of his diagnosis, unknowingly, my father increased his financial risks. And he compounded his vulnerability by keeping his diagnosis a secret. Usually, he asked my brother and me before he made major decisions in his life. But this time, he asked our opinion without divulging the most important piece of information that may have made us look deeper into, why now.

In the early winter of 2013, I got a call from my father while in Florida. He wanted to ask my opinion about marrying Marie.

My father said, "She's a good person. I love her and I'm thinking I would sell the house and move to the Cape."

I listened to him with apprehension as he told me. It baffled me. Why now? But I could never dictate how my father should live his life or with whom he should live it.

It didn't sit right with me at first, and not with my brother either. Despite my father's previous adamant opposition, he made a sudden shift in his life plan. Suddenly, he wanted to commit to marriage and selling his home.

I said, "If it's what you want, Dad. I'm okay with it if this makes you happy."

I gave him my blessing, and so did my brother. My father planned to have a prenup agreement. Marriage wouldn't change his feelings about keeping his finances separate, which he always had. I didn't presume that Alzheimer's played a role in his decision to create a will and other long-term care directives. He had established these long ago. I remember from the age of thirteen, when my parents asked me to choose a guardian in case they died. In my twenties, after my mother died, my father updated his directives and appointed me as his proxy. The beneficiaries of his will back then were my brother and I split 50/50, and he made it known that is what he wanted in the future. His marriage to Marie wouldn't change his long-term decisions.

LESSONS LEARNED

I had no idea how impaired my father's judgment was, but Marie did. On October 4, 2013, Mass General Hospital's medical records revealed Marie reported to my father's physician that she first noticed difficulties two to three years prior. She described my father as having a hard time registering and remembering information, and his inability to handle finances. Six days later, on October 10, 2013, Marie was with him when he signed his directive giving me power of attorney to handle his finances. Yet she acted against his wishes, took over financial control, and combined his money with hers. And she kept all of this information to herself. I only discovered this on January 31, 2025.

There is no good reason and no benefit to keeping an Alzheimer's diagnosis a secret. Even the shortest duration of time can create an opportunity for financial abuse, coercion, and exploitation.

The two initial steps to protect the finances and medical choices of the person diagnosed with Alzheimer's are:

> Step 1. Disclose the Alzheimer's diagnosis to loved ones and close family within days, not weeks.
>
> Step 2. Contact a social worker and begin the process of decision-making. Potential advocates, family, and loved ones need to be present. Use Facetime or Zoom if necessary.

"The perpetrators of predatory financial abuse do sometimes work for several days — or longer — to establish a relationship with a vulnerable older person. Whereas predators are purposefully out to defraud or exploit others, opportunists are those who end up financially exploiting an older person because...well, the opportunity arose, usually due to a relationship between the older person and the one who ends up exploiting the situation. Such 'opportunistic' abuse can be committed by family members, paid in-home care providers, or even trusted people outside the home, such as financial advisors or spiritual advisors. (Of course, suspicion or resentment of an older person's new relationship does not always mean that abuse or even manipulative situations are occurring.)"[20]

"Exploitation in the context of personal relationships is often especially tricky for families to address. The older person may be quite attached to – or otherwise feel dependent on – the person that others perceive as suspicious or problematic. Or there may be concerns about stirring up family dramas and conflicts, by voicing concerns about a sibling or another relative. People are often unsure of what exactly constitutes illegal activity, and what can be done if they are concerned about financial exploitation."[21] From Better Health While Aging, Practical Information for Aging Health & Caregivers, Financial Exploitation in Aging: What to Know & What to Do, by Leslie Kernisan, MD, MPH.

The Progression

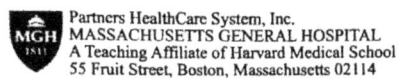
Partners HealthCare System, Inc.
MASSACHUSETTS GENERAL HOSPITAL
A Teaching Affiliate of Harvard Medical School
55 Fruit Street, Boston, Massachusetts 02114

MRN: 1510213 (MGH)
SULLIVAN SR, JOHN J
Date of Birth: 03/05/1939
Sex: M

Notes from 1/1/2011 through 4/1/2016 (cont)

3   PAC Report   Final   Sherman, Janet ...

Patient: SULLIVAN SR, JOHN J 1510213(MGH) 03/05/39 M
Author: Electronically Signed by Janet C Sherman, Phd

Signed 10/24/2013 15:15
Visit Date: 10/04/2013

Psychology Assessment Center
Boston, MA 02114-2696

Tel. (617) 724-5439
FAX (617) 724-3726

NEUROPSYCHOLOGICAL EVALUATION

SULLIVAN, John
MRN: 1510213
DOB: 3/5/39
DOE: 10/4/13

Reason for referral:
Mr. John Sullivan is a 74 year old right-handed gentleman referred by Dr. Deborah Blacker of the MGH Memory Disorders Unit. Mr. Sullivan is a retired firefighter who presents with family concerns about progressive difficulties with memory. Dr. Blacker's impression based on her 6/17/13 evaluation is Mild Cognitive Impairment, with primary or sole deficits in memory. He was referred for this evaluation to provide information regarding current cognitive functioning and to help address etiology of difficulties. The current evaluation consisted of a clinical interview with Mr. Sullivan and his wife, review of the relevant medical record and administration of a battery of neuropsychological tests. Informed consent for this evaluation was obtained from Mr. Sullivan that indicated his understanding of the purpose of the evaluation and limits of confidentiality and a signed consent form is in his internal record.

History of presenting problem
Mrs. Sullivan reports that she first started noticing difficulties two to three years ago, and reports that they have progressed very gradually. He was evaluated by a physician in Florida in January 2013 for memory difficulties. An MRI indicated bilateral small vessel ischemic changes. Based on that evaluation, he was thought to have prodromal AD and was started on Aricept. At today's evaluation, Mr. Sullivan states that he is "scared about Alzheimer's" and "wants to be on top of things."
Mr. Sullivan reports that he doesn't really notice any difficulties with memory. However, his wife reports that she has to tell him things at least three times before he gets it. She was initially unsure if his difficulties were related to poor hearing, but she has found that his difficulties extend beyond this. For example, he looks puzzled even when he can hear her, and is slower to learn new information, taking six weeks to learn their new zip code after a move in August. She describes her husband as having a hard time both registering and remembering information; they report that reminders and cues are helpful. They also report some increased difficulty with routes and directions. When they first moved to the Cape he had a hard time learning a simple route, though now that he has learned it, he remembers it. He is the primary driver and uses a GPS which his wife programs for him. They are always together when he goes out. He has not had any accidents, but by his wife's report, he weaves a little on the road and she sometimes gets nervous when he drives onto the rumble strip. They report that he has always had difficulty with names. He denies difficulty understanding speech, although his hearing can interfere. He reads without difficulty and follows the news. He was able to relate information regarding the Affordable Care Act and Government Shut Down. He knew about sports events in Boston but had a hard time naming the team that the Red Sox were facing in the playoffs. They report that he is less mechanical than in the past, with Mr. Sullivan stating that he has "lost his edge." His wife reports that it takes him a while to get from A to B and he has had some difficulty with recent financial decisions. They also describe increased difficulty with multi-tasking, though Mr. Sullivan reports that his concentration has always been poor and that he has always had a tendency to do things too quickly. His wife reports that if he gets distracted or interrupted he has difficulty getting back on track and she feels that this is worse than in the past. He describes himself as organized and indicates no change. They deny change in behavior, social interactions, or personality. They report a longstanding tendency to over react when he gets angry, and state that this happens mainly around driving. While he has always had a temper, they state that he is more in control of it now.
Regarding ADL's, Mr. Sullivan continues to drive, as above. He manages his own medications, though he sometimes gets confused about whether he has taken his morning medications. He keeps all of his medications in a plastic bag, which he states works well for him. They recently combined their finances and she is in the process of taking them over. She reports that he was getting the bills paid though not always correctly. She also reports that she finds previously paid bills in "weird places".

Page 1 of 9

Record obtained by Jacqueline from Mass General Hospital medical records on January 31, 2025.
From medical records collected by author

Chapter 7
Why the Sudden Change of Heart?

Alzheimer's created a tug-of-war between my father's strength and his growing fears. My father's decision to keep the diagnosis a secret between him and Marie was a colossal miscalculation of his judgment. This is a hallmark of this disease.

The fact is the person who has the capacity in the relationship becomes more influential when the other person in the relationship has Alzheimer's. This influence can be positive, nurturing, and major support, but there also is a grim reality where the opposite can be true.

My father's life was falling apart. He was not functioning with 100 percent clarity, and that made him extremely vulnerable. Because of the disease, the balance between my father and Marie shifted. Marie became his only confidant and sounding board. By default, she had the power to persuade. While my father's future unraveled, Marie gained his complete trust. I know my father never wanted to be a burden to us. And the thought of a nursing home scared him to death. It terrified him. And Marie knew it.

Before being diagnosed with Alzheimer's, my father was consistent in his decisions, including his declaration, *I'll die before I ever leave my house.* However, six months after his Alzheimer's diagnosis, he put his home on the market. He never wanted to sell his home, he never wanted to get married, and he never wanted to move to the Cape. There was only one variable that changed "never" to "happening" and that was Alzheimer's.

I went to my father's home one afternoon to help him pack and look through some things he wanted to give me. Marie was there that day.

I said, "Marie, can you believe Dad is selling his home, moving to the Cape, and you're getting married?"

She looked at me with a joyous grin that showed her whitened teeth.

Marie said, "I never thought it would happen."

She was right. It would never have happened if my father did not have Alzheimer's. We packed our memories and removed them from the place where I grew up, and my parents' first home. They worked hard to achieve their dream of owning it and the bond they shared etched itself into every corner and it remained even after her death.

When my father began cycling to raise money for cancer, he hung a shadow box above our stairway in the hall. In it, he pinned the medals he accumulated over the years from walks and rides in my mother's memory. From every finish line my father crossed, the medals he received revealed his love for my mother and the disease that took her away. When he packed them, he took one down at a time, and with such reverence, he folded the attached ribbon around the medal and laid them in a box.

Both my mother and father kept things that connected them to their past. They displayed them as reminders to never forget who they were and where they came from. They were invaluable to them and that made it tough to choose what we saved and what we gave away. There were so many everyday items that held a story, like the wooden thermometer that had hung in our kitchen since the 1970s.

It was the first year of a not-so-good wood stove during the energy crisis. The Franklin was an innovative stove with a major hidden flaw. The design of the flue reduced its efficiency. For the stove to burn throughout the night, the draft had to remain open. That meant if you closed the draft, the fire would smother and go out at night. My father tried to best to make it work. He filled it up before bed and had the stove roaring. It grew so hot one night that it glowed red and buckled the back plate inside the stove. But by the time morning came, for the umpteenth time, the fire burned out again. Not a single ember was left to start a fire.

My brother and I knew it was going to be a bitter and cold night when my mother left the faucets on a drip before we went to bed.

Fear Knocked — Jacqueline Sullivan Wyco

Remarkably, we never had a frozen pipe. Some mornings while my brother and I ate breakfast we saw our breath. We didn't need the thermometer to show how cold it was. My mother was always up before the sun. You could hear her downstairs as she started her routine. First, she opened the damper on the stove. The cast iron plate squealed as it turned. Then the crumpling of newspapers followed. On school days, I always knew what time it was by the crack of kindling and the cinders that blew up with the loud rush of air through the stovepipe in my closet. I never used an alarm clock. I didn't need one.

We packed that thermometer, like so many things in our home, as if it were a priceless treasure. That seemed to bother Marie, and that's putting it mildly. More than once, she expressed her aversion to our things and our home.

Marie said, "I would never live here."

And I understood that in a way, it wasn't her home, but I don't think she even wanted to make it her own. Overall, I liked Marie. I believed she wanted to be part of our family. But Marie never shared intimate details about her past like we did. We were open with Marie. We talked about ourselves, our past, and our childhood experiences. But Marie, not so much.

In the twenty-one years I got to know Marie, I heard very few stories about her parents, growing up with them, and her siblings. She didn't talk about raising her children. Whatever happened in Marie's family is not my business. And it's not for me to put out there in this book. Everyone has a right to privacy. This was different. It's hard to explain. But there was a side to Marie she didn't let anyone see. Sometimes she slipped, and when I saw her in these split seconds, I got the feeling, she despised us.

Marie watched and helped pack as we sorted out our belongings. She was in her glory and eager to begin her new life as it came closer to fruition. Marie had her opinions on what to keep. I expected it, as she and my father would be married and living together. Marie's comments were general. They fell in line with what everyone says and goes through when they move.

She said to my father, "I don't want that. Why do you need that? There's no room for that. Maybe Jacqueline would take it or John."

Why the Sudden Change of Heart?

But that was until my father asked if I wanted a distinct silver platter. Before my father could finish his sentence, Marie interrupted. I remember her face as she sneered.

She said, "That's not real silver. It's silver plate, not worth anything."

Her comment lingered, and I felt the slight jab aimed at my mother. I didn't respond. Neither did my father.

It took weeks for my father to pack, and my brother and I helped as often as we could. We helped him clean out the attic above our garage. My father made a comment that made me stop and wonder if there was something else going on with him. I was at the back of my brother's truck, standing next to my father at the tailgate.

He said, "I could never leave this for you guys to deal with."

My father said it in a way that made me think he had a terminal disease. My thoughts went from, *does he know?* To, *no, he wouldn't keep this to himself.* Then I thought, *but what if he is dying and he's not telling me?* I kept moving, and the thoughts cycled back and forth in my head. He looked healthy. He was planning his future. My father remained composed and focused, and I took his lead, shifting my attention to the monumental task of packing.

I could have brought it up and told him it's never too late to change your mind. I could have reassured him and told him whatever it was, whatever was happening, we could work it out, and we would deal with any problem he had. But I didn't. I dismissed what I was feeling and remained silent. It bothers me to this day. Why didn't I stop, pull him to the side, and ask him what was truly going on?

LESSONS LEARNED

I believe my father's fears drove him to make the hardest decisions of his life. He also didn't want to burden us with caring for him or leave us with the enormity of sorting through our childhood home. Alzheimer's was an opportunity for Marie to fulfill her desires. I believe she consoled him and settled his fears and terrors with a promise. Her commitment to stand by him in sickness and in health convinced him that his marriage to her, selling his home, and moving to the Cape, was his best answer to living out the rest of his life with Alzheimer's.

Having a social worker from the onset of diagnosis to mediate advocates, family, and loved ones, can help the person with Alzheimer's in four ways.

1. Evaluation. An Alzheimer's diagnosis comes with many decisions to make. An experienced social worker can help advocates, family, and loved ones, look at and discuss all possible solutions, not just one.

2. Communication through mediation. The structure of mediation gives the person with Alzheimer's, advocates, family members, and loved ones a supportive environment where all can speak and be heard. The power of persuasion is neutralized. Decisions by the person with Alzheimer's can be made without feeling cornered or pressured by one person's beliefs and opinions on what they should do. These meetings support everyone.

3. Documentation through routine mediation protects the decisions of a person with Alzheimer's through validation. Mediation keeps everyone up to date on the changing needs of the person. Ultimately, these meetings will strengthen, protect, and reinforce the person's financial, medical, and personal decisions.

4. The byproduct of these group meetings is transparency. And transparency naturally creates a system of checks and balances which reduces the risk of financial loss, questionable changes to medical, or long-term decisions, extortion, abuse, and neglect.

Chapter 8

First Came Alzheimer's, Then Came Marriage

My father married Marie in July 2013, six months after his Alzheimer's diagnosis. At seventy-four years old, my father's memory was failing, and Marie chose to marry him despite what my father's future held. Marie kept the secret, although she could have decided to share it with me and my brother before she married my father.

    Marie planned an intimate wedding. With two phone calls, she completed what took me months to accomplish on my own wedding. In less time than it took me to walk down the boardwalk to the beach for my ceremony, Marie booked the justice of the peace, chose vows, and the venue for their wedding and the reception. She decided, for the wedding bands, they would use a ring my father already had and the engagement ring he bought for her with three diamonds that signified the past, present, and future.

    Marie called the minister who married my brother, and his wife, and asked if she could perform her ceremony. She also booked the same inn on the Cape where I had planned my wedding and reserved rooms for my family. Most brides, no matter their age, and regardless of how extravagant or simple the ceremony, integrate personal touches that reflect meaning. But Marie chose to create her wedding by recreating the elements from my wedding and my brother's. She included the details even down to the pouring of the sand. The same ritual my brother- and sister-in-law performed after they exchanged rings.

    My father's Alzheimer's became concealed behind his union with Marie. For some reason, I took my attention off my father and stopped wondering where his change of heart came from. However, I don't know of one person at their ceremony, including Marie's family, who knew my father had Alzheimer's. It appeared to me that their partnership was equal. However, due to my father's cognitive decline, becoming Mrs. John J. Sullivan automatically came with all the control of decision-making in their relationship.

⸘⸘⸘

In my adult years, after my mother died, and before Marie entered the picture, my father and I spent a lot of time together. Since my mother died, my father and I grew close. I called my father if I needed a pick-me-up. If I was down about a problem, he'd help me find the answer. I always felt better after I talked to him. He could pull me out of a mood and make me laugh within minutes. There were countless times throughout my years as an adult, we said what the other was thinking. When I called him, often he said, "I was just thinking about you."

Sometimes, we'd go to the North End in Boston for lunch, then cross over to Haymarket and Faneuil Hall to go shopping at Filene's and Jordan's on Washington Street for the afternoon. Other times, we'd take a drive down towards Marshfield to hit a few consignment stores along the route where my mother used to go. We weren't just father and daughter. We were more like friends.

If I had a day off, I'd call to ask if he wanted to grab lunch or something. My father always said yes, but since 2011, two years before his marriage to Marie, our one-on-one time slowly disappeared. Nine times out of ten, she came. She was either with him or met us on her lunch break. Marie always wore that same smile when we greeted each other. She appeared to be affectionate, laid back, and easygoing. Occasionally, she sprung for lunch, and when she did, it convinced me that she wasn't taking advantage of my father. She showed me what I wanted to see in a partner for my father and over time, she diffused any doubt I had about her feelings for my father. I wondered about her motives in the past, but those, too, subsided.

In 2011, after I married Mark, we moved to Hubbardston, a more rural town, two hours from the Berkshires, and fifteen miles outside of Worcester. My father and Marie continued to visit me and stay over as they did on the Cape before I met Mark. At the time, my father was still living in my childhood home and Marie was in her condo on the North Shore. Our home in Hubbardston backed up to the forest. It abutted acres of conservation land with trails, ponds, and streams. My father called our house the bed-and-breakfast.

My father sold his home on July 22, 2013. Mark and I didn't think twice about inviting him and Marie to stay with us while they were looking for their new place. They were easy-going as a couple. My father was upbeat. I loved being around him.

On days when my father and Marie weren't looking at houses, they hung out with me and Mark. Mostly they enjoyed sitting on the swing chair on the back deck. They sipped coffee, read the paper, and enjoyed the sun and the quiet. Mark and I gave them a key, and they came and went as they pleased. At night after supper, my father watched baseball and had his tea while Marie had her wine. She watched the game and looked content sitting by my father while we chatted with her about whatever came up. It was relaxing, and they both felt at home. I still wasn't aware of my father's Alzheimer's diagnosis at this time. Although he stalled mid-sentence and struggled to find the right word at times, I didn't pay close attention. Marie filled in the gaps so effortlessly that my father appeared more cognizant than he really was.

They found a place on the Cape in the town where I used to live. They moved into their home in the middle of October that year. And about a month after settling into their condo, Marie mentioned they were looking for a new primary care doctor, closer to them. I referred her to a physician who was my client when I had my practice on the Cape. She was new to the area and was building her practice at the community wellness center. I gave her name and number to Marie. When I followed up with Marie, she said the physician wasn't taking on new patients. I thought it was kind of strange not to be taking on any new patients so soon. However, Marie informed me of the primary care physician she chose. It was one with whom I had no connection.

It wouldn't be long till she and my father were off again to Florida for the winter. Before they left, Marie made their reservations to return home for Christmas, their usual routine. For years, Marie and my father had spent every Christmas Eve with her family, and every Christmas Day with Mark, me, and our family at our house. Soon after the new year, my father and Marie returned to Florida. On New Year's Eve 2013, my father became a grandfather when my brother John and sister-in-law Karen had their firstborn. He was thrilled when my brother asked him how he would feel if they named her Beverly, after my mother.

My brother and I talked to my father often throughout the winter. Marie was always in the background on speaker, adding to the conversation about what she had scheduled for the day. Usually, she remarked on where they were going to eat and if they had been to the beach or down to the pool. Their social calendar was always busy. They played cards and went to almost every event at the clubhouse. I felt reassured by Marie. Her remarks made it sound as if they were both doing well. However, I missed my father when he was gone. Each year, they stayed longer in Florida and eventually moved out their date to come home to mid-June. Summers flew by and between work and the two-hour drive each way to their home on the Cape, our time together was short.

In 2014 and 2015, our visits were more spread out, and my father's cognitive decline became more noticeable to me when we talked. I noticed my father called Marie, *Sis*, my mother's nickname. Sometimes, my father caught it and corrected himself, but sometimes he didn't. Marie let it go, and so did I. But Marie hinted at a problem one afternoon while I was watching a ball game with my father when he went to the bathroom.

Marie said, "Your father does the strangest things."

I said, "Like what?"

She watched to see if my father was on the way back from the bathroom.

She said, "He put his dirty dishes in the bathroom sink."

I said nothing, I just listened.

Marie dropped a hint and let it ride. Her comment stayed with me, and I sat in the worry that my father's confusion was more than a memory lapse. While visiting on another day with my father, he mentioned he'd like to take a trip to New York to see the memorial of 9/11. He wanted us all to go. As he was talking, he stopped in mid-sentence and his hand trembled.

My father said, "In the fall."

He stopped again.

Then he said, "Summer?"

It was already late summer in 2014, but he couldn't distinguish a timeline. I made light of it, brushed it off, and reasoned it out.

I said, "It's easy to get mixed up because in Florida it must seem like one season all year round." Leaving him that day, I couldn't stop thinking about what happened, and when I pulled into my garage, Mark was there. I broke down.

I said, "There's something wrong with my father. I don't know if it's maybe dementia."

It wasn't long after that I learned of my father's diagnosis. My husband and I were visiting him and Marie. All of us were sitting at the kitchen table, and I asked if anyone wanted to take a walk. They chose to stay home and hang out. When I returned, I walked in to find a solemness in the room that I hadn't experienced in years, since my mother died. I didn't know it, but my father had told Mark the devastating news while I was gone. Marie and my father asked Mark if they should tell me. I'm not sure where the idea of keeping the diagnosis from me came from. They never sat my brother and his wife down either. Understanding the dynamics of my father's relationship with Marie and his mental state as I do now, I can only guess. When I looked at my father's face, I knew it was serious.

"What's the matter?" I asked.

He said, "Sit down, I have to tell you something."

I thought maybe he had cancer, and in my mind, that was no big deal. He could survive cancer. My husband was sitting to his left and Marie sat with her back toward me, facing my father. I didn't look at her. All I saw was my husband's eyes fill up.

He said, "I have Alzheimer's."

He choked back the tears and hugged me tight. He held on and the weight of his body rested on mine and, as he sobbed, he sank deeper into my arms.

I said, "Dad, don't worry, I'll take care of you. You can come to my house when you need more help."

I saw Marie when I went to sit down. Her eyes bulged when she looked at me. She leaned forward and blasted out.

"What, you're going to change his diapers? He's a big guy, and he has depression."

I couldn't look at my father when she said it. She didn't shed a tear. Her eyes never welled up. Now, I know this news wasn't a shock to her. She knew for two years and ten months what I had just found out. It wasn't until I said I'd take care of him that she flew off the handle. She lost her temper. Then she tried to discourage me from caring for him and belittled him in front of me. Her response made no sense.

Later, my husband told me she smirked when my father told me he had Alzheimer's. I thought *she couldn't have. Maybe he had misread her. We were grieving, we were stunned and at a loss for what came next. What would provoke such a reaction?*

My husband and I were trying to process what my father had told us, and what that meant for him going forward. Marie, without skipping a beat, spun us around. She fast-forwarded us to the end with vivid imagery of my father sitting in a diaper. And me, struggling to change him. Marie took our torn hearts and shredded them. Without a breath of hesitation, she conjured the vision and rubbed our faces into the grim future. It was a place we couldn't bring ourselves to go.

My father stopped crying.

He said, "Enough of that."

He turned to me.

"I'm going to fight this thing."

He pounded the table with his fist like a gavel. There wasn't a cure, but he wanted to live. He said if there were a medical trial, he would do it. If it couldn't help him, he said it may help someone else after him.

My father said, "I kept it to myself because I couldn't accept it."

In October 2015, thirty-four months had passed since his Alzheimer's diagnosis.

Marie said, "Your father is on a med that slows the progression."

My father knew he was going to die from a disease that had no cure. But the thought of ending up in a nursing home terrified him more than anything. He responded to calls to the fire department in the era of widespread nursing home abuse during the 1970s and early 1980s.

Some nursing homes were senior facilities, others were old homes that were turned into nursing homes. These places gave him nightmares. He told me stories of dozens of helpless, sick, and disoriented residents. They were lying on cots and dorm-like beds shoved in close to one another in a single room that used to be the living room or dining room. Some were crying, others were moaning. The smell of urine burned the inside of his nose, and some lay in their feces that covered the sheets. Some walked around naked, and none were let out. The neglect was heartbreaking. It's what my father called a real-life horror show. The elder care system had been in a state of full-fledged disrepair. It was a crime against humanity. That's the nursing home my father connected with in his mind, and that's why I told him I would take care of him.

My father gave me a high sign and pointed to the desk drawer where he kept his paperwork, while Marie talked to Mark. I didn't bring up anything that day regarding legal matters. I knew I was his power of attorney, health care proxy, and executor of his will. He and Marie both had separate trusts in which their residence on the Cape was in. I was my father's trustee, and my brother the alternate. Marie chose her advocates and trustees of her half of the Cape condo. Marie attended all my father's doctor's appointments. From now on I believed Marie would inform me.

I had no discussion with my father about when I should begin as his advocate. I am not sure if the physicians told Marie the importance of invoking his power of attorney, but no one communicated with me. Somewhere in the back of my mind, I had the impression that his physicians would let me know. When they didn't, I continued to wait. In doing so, I jeopardized every legal decision my father made.

I put my trust and blind faith in Marie, my father's legal documents, and the medical and legal systems. I should have taken a day and gone over every detail with my father, Marie, my brother, and our spouses. By not taking this first step, I gave Marie an unobstructed path to my father's medical and financial decision-making. Marie was in the driver's seat, and I put her there.

LESSONS LEARNED

My father protected his finances, assets, and medical decisions with advanced directives. This single, one-layered security on paper wasn't nearly enough protection. I've learned that a person with Alzheimer's needs a comprehensive long-term defensive strategy that requires multiple layers of protection.

Have you ever heard of the Swiss cheese model of security?

"The risk of a threat becoming a reality is mitigated by the differing layers and types of defenses that are —"layered"— behind each other. Therefore, in theory, lapses and weaknesses in one defense do not allow a risk to materialize (e.g. a hole in each slice in the stack aligning with holes in all other slices), since other defenses also exist (e.g. other slices of cheese), to prevent a single point of failure."[22] From Wikipedia, the article entitled "Swiss Cheese Model."

Your first layer of security: Disclose the diagnosis.

Your second layer of security: Enlist a social worker as part of the person's care team. Routine communication, and documentation, are critical and powerful methods of protection, as you will understand more throughout this book.

Chapter 9
Things Aren't Always What They Appear

In 2015, my father was seventy-six years old. Marie shadowed my father and monitored his conversations with me when I called. She corrected him when he confused details and helped him finish his thoughts. And when he stalled mid-sentence, she prompted him. I talked with my father two or three times a week, when he was at home and while he was in Florida. Often it was to say hi, nothing important, but every time he called me, or I called him, Marie was in the background on speaker. She listened closely and always answered before my father responded to my questions. *Hi Dad, how are you?* He followed her lead and repeated after her. — *We're good, how about you?*— Marie cued and completed my father's sentences. Over time, she became my father's voice and his decision-maker.

During this time, my father couldn't follow the navigation on his GPS. He could not listen to it, follow its instructions and make turns in enough time. He confused left and right and this made it impossible for him to walk or drive anywhere alone. His medical records indicated on August 7, 2015, "He drives and has not had any accidents, but occasionally he gets lost, even on familiar routes."

When my father called me from Florida to tell me he bought a new car, I wondered how he compared prices, searched for the dealer, and negotiated the deal during this stage of his disease. The car salesman at the dealership most likely didn't pick up on his cognitive decline. He had no idea that over two years had passed since my father's initial diagnosis of Alzheimer's.

It wasn't unusual for my father to buy a new car. He had bought

Fear Knocked — Jacqueline Sullivan Wyco

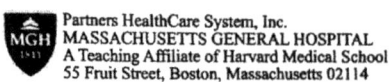

Medical record obtained by Jacqueline from Mass General Hospital on January 31, 2025. *From records collected by the author*

new vehicles in the past, traded them in, and upgraded them over the years. He took great care of them. But purchasing a car is daunting for the person who has a healthy brain. In talking with my father during this time, by the end of one sentence, he couldn't repeat three words that were said. Yet, he was able to purchase a brand-new car with his level of impairment.

My father drove when Mark and I visited him in Florida that year. He took us to the Audubon Sanctuary near their condo one day. But Marie got us there by instructing my father where to drive, when to turn, and where to park. My father got lost coming out of the restroom just a few minutes after we parked. Mark and I were standing on the boardwalk with Marie waiting for him when she told us when they were there before he went out the wrong door. There were two. One was off the boardwalk where we were and the other opened inside the educational hut. Marie kept an eye out for him and looked around the corner.

Marie said, "I have to watch him."

Mark walked in to check on him, and sure enough, he went out through the door inside.

During my visit, Marie and I walked to Walmart. She brought up a discussion as if she were thinking out loud.

She said, "I'm wondering when I'll have to choose where we live. The Cape or Florida? What do you think?"

I said, "I don't know."

She said, "I'm not sure, maybe we'll sell the Cape and live here."

I didn't say anything else, because I thought, *where did this idea come from? It didn't come from my father before Alzheimer's, and he didn't mention it after his diagnosis. But now Marie had floated the idea of permanently moving to Florida.*

As my conversation continued with Marie, I approached the subject of taking over and paying my father's bills, and since their finances were separate, there should have been no issue.

I said, "Marie, I can take care of my father's bills."

But she immediately and politely declined. "I'll let you know if it gets too much. Right now, I'm fine. It's no trouble."

I grew more uncertain why Marie had thought of moving permanently to Florida.

LESSON LEARNED

Marie's pattern of control gradually intensified with my father's decline. It wasn't difficult for Marie to influence my father. It was easy for her since his mind was deteriorating. I didn't understand what coercion was and I never heard of coercive control until I began studying my father, his disease, and his relationship with Marie. The signs were subtle. "In coercive control, the abuser seeks to isolate the victim. The abuser will use tactics, such as limiting access to money or monitoring all communication, as a controlling effort."[23] "Coercive control is a gradual, subtle form of domestic abuse that entraps their victim in a hostage-like situation."[24] From Healthline, "Coercive Control: 12 Signs and How to Get Out."

My father gave me legal permission to move him, and he also should have documented it in his power of attorney, which state he wanted to reside in when the disease made it too difficult for him to travel between two residences. Especially, if ever I needed to prove his intentions in court.

As the disease progressed in 2016, my father became more obsessive. I got a frantic phone call from him one afternoon. He was positive that someone had stolen all his money. In the background, Marie said no, it didn't happen, rejecting his claim. My father was persistent and told me he needed to call the police and the FBI. My father grew hypervigilant about the safety of his money. Marie followed me on a separate call. She informed me of his ongoing compulsion to check and recheck the whereabouts of his money and wallet. Part of this obsessive compulsion stemmed from the disease, but I wondered if his imagined narrative was in reality, a moment of clarity.

At seventy-seven years old, my father was in the middle stage of Alzheimer's, the space where delusion intruded his mind. I got a call from him about 11 o'clock. I was already in bed. "Dad Home" came up on my iPhone screen and when I answered, I heard Marie's voice in the background.

She said to my father, "Hang up the phone. She's probably in bed. It's too late, Jacqueline and Mark go to bed early."

He didn't say hi to me yet. He was listening to Marie. When she realized I was on the phone, she quickly apologized for calling so late.

I said, "You're not bothering me, Dad. You can call me anytime. Don't be sorry. Marie, it's fine. No need to apologize."

My father usually asked me how I was at first, but this call was different. He wanted to know if I had seen his deceased mother.

I said, "I haven't, but if I do, I will have her call you."

My father said, "Oh. I want to talk to her. You haven't seen her?"

He was on a mission. I could not change the subject, and I didn't want to tell him she had died.

"If I see her, I'll tell her to call you, Dad."

He felt reassured and we both said *I love you*, then goodnight. My head was swimming. His past fused with the present and as the weeks went by, there would be more confusion and more forgetfulness. But when darkness set in, his longing to connect to his mother grew stronger.

I reached out to Marie the following day and told her I wanted to go to his appointment with the Alzheimer's physician when they came home. My father was in the thick of it. Alzheimer's created a duality. My father was not his disease, yet the disease was turning him into a version of himself who was unrecognizable.

LESSONS LEARNED

My father was suffering from sundowning. "A group of behaviors, feelings, and thoughts people who have Alzheimer's or dementia can experience as the sun sets. The behaviors start or get worse around sunset or sundown. However, this delirium can potentially occur at any time, not just at sunset." [25] From the Cleveland Clinic,"Sundown Syndrome: Causes, Treatment & Symptoms."

Chapter 10
A Fragile State Teetering on Volatile

It was the middle of June 2016, and my father and Marie returned home from Florida. I went down to visit a week after they returned. Shortly after I arrived, my father picked up his car keys to make a quick run to the market, and I tagged along. It was close enough to walk. By car, all my father needed to do was drive to the traffic light at the entrance of the condo community and go straight across the road into the parking lot. But he went left instead of straight and couldn't figure out where to turn. On the way home, he went to a different exit and drove through two stop signs.

Before Alzheimer's, I considered my father an exceptional driver. My father responded to numerous car accidents and fatalities during his firefighter career. When he used the jaws of life to extract trapped victims, it was a vivid reminder to stay defensive behind the wheel.

Alzheimer's warped his judgment and delayed his response time. After we were back at his place, I talked with Marie about what happened and told her I was worried about him driving. But Marie was already aware. My father's medical records from Mass General Hospital dated ten months prior, August 7, 2015, determined that my father's safety was at risk in terms of driving and the physician recommended to Marie that my father undergo a driving evaluation back then. Marie never mentioned any of this. In response to my concerns, she recounted an incident over the weekend where he nearly caused an accident.

Marie said, "Me and my daughter were in the car at the rotary and your father came up on the turn-off when he kept going. We yelled, turn here, and he had passed the turn already and he tried to make it anyway. He jerked the wheel and almost collided with another car."

My father couldn't remember the way home. Marie told me it wasn't the first time. His brain couldn't process left from right, and his reaction time had significantly dropped.

Marie said, "Your father has an appointment coming up with his doctor. I'll talk to him about it."

I didn't know, but Marie had changed Alzheimer's physicians. She called a day or so after his appointment.

She said, "The doctor recommended your father go for a driving test."

And when he did, it confirmed that he shouldn't be driving. That didn't go over well with my father, and there was no easy way to make him understand that his ability to go where he wanted, when he wanted, under his own volition, would be removed. It was inevitable, because of the disease, but it was a jarring realization each time he had to be reminded of why he couldn't get in his car and drive. His level of impairment only made the situation worse.

The doctor advised Marie to confiscate his keys. Marie reminded my father why she took them after he asked her where they were. It confused him. And when reasoning with him stopped working, he grew agitated, so much so that Marie called me.

Marie said, "Your father is upset. He wants his keys. When I reminded him, he got angry and yelled he wanted them, NOW!"

I asked Marie to put him on the phone.

I said, "Dad, you can't drive anymore. You took a driving test, and you didn't pass it. I'm sorry, I know you want to drive."

He seemed to settle down, but when we hung up, it was only a few minutes later before Marie called again. She reminded my father, and his level of agitation grew.

He said, "I want my keys. I want my car."

He was laser-focused, and I could almost feel his adrenalin pumping through the phone with the vibration of his voice. He was at a critical point, and I needed help.

I paced on the front porch as I talked to my father. I never expected trying to calm him would have the opposite effect. Reasoning with him provoked him even further. I knew that people with Alzheimer's can lash out. The aim of my discussion immediately turned to his safety. My father never grew violent in the past, and I wanted to prevent that from happening. Both my husband and I recommended to Marie that she distance herself from him, even if that meant going outside.

I told her I'd contact his Alzheimer's doctor and call her right back. Mark had gone inside. Marie talked as I walked into the house.

Marie said, "If your father becomes physical, I'll just call the police."

Mark overheard her.

Mark said, "Marie, please go in another room, or even outside if you have to but distance yourself from him for your safety and his."

We asked Marie multiple times to separate herself from my father, but she didn't. This situation had already escalated. Marie, with her continual engagement, fueled an existing inferno. I heard him shout in the background.

I repeated, "Marie, please distance yourself and give me a chance to call his doctor."

I got off the phone with Marie and immediately called his Alzheimer's physician, who was a board-certified specialist with over thirty-five years of experience in neurodegenerative disorders. It was a Sunday morning of a holiday weekend, and his voicemail directed me to an answering service. He was away in another country, and I was told by the answering service that I could speak with the doctor on call. I told her I was not interested and that I needed to speak with his doctor because he was familiar with his case, and his meds, and my father needed help now.

His doctor called me within minutes. He recommended my father take an additional tablet of medication he was already on. I called Marie and gave her the doctor's instructions and within a half hour, my father settled down. Because of my experience, I recommend caregivers speak to the person's physician to create a plan of action before a crisis. Find out what you can do to de-escalate and calm the person if ever a situation like this arises. Ask about what medication and dosage they'd recommend.

Despite the effectiveness of the medication, he felt completely drained. My father had experienced a prolonged duration of acute stress, where stress hormones were released into his bloodstream. His anxiety triggered the Fight or Flight response. But his Alzheimer's had deteriorated his ability to accurately perceive danger, or a threatening situation. I perceived taking away my father's keys as non-threatening, an act intended to keep him and others safe. But he perceived taking away his keys as a threat. And each time we explained why we took away his keys, his response heightened and intensified with each reminder.

During the moderate stage of this disease, my father had lost the wherewithal to interpret logic and reasoning, and taking his keys away made no sense to him. He perceived it as a threatening gesture. To him, this decision came out of left field without warning, and he saw it as an attack. Anxiety is pain and taking away my father's car keys so late in his disease caused immense frustration and anxiety. I suggest this be a topic of discussion early in the disease because I know we could have done a better job of managing this situation to prevent his pain.

LESSONS LEARNED

I suggest you talk to the Alzheimer's physician about agitation medications before you need them. I advise you to speak with a social worker trained in dementia to create a list of strategies for diffusing agitation and stressful situations. A dosage of medication or strategy that is effective in de-escalating a situation once may not work for the next.

What to do when a dementia patient is aggressive or escalating.

- Don't argue or use negative words like —"No"— or —"You can't"—. This can be challenging, but it's critical that a person doesn't perceive you as combative or a barrier.
- Even if you're right, don't try to prove it. This is just another way of saying they're wrong, which can make them agitated.
- Avoid aggressive body language, like clenching your fists, crossing arms, or scowling.
- Maintain eye contact, but don't stare aggressively.

- Speak firmly and calmly.
- If they're family, say something that triggers the relationship, like, —"Dad, I understand you want to do X. I can help." — Otherwise, use their first name.
- Keep your voice low and modulated.
- Try to release or undo whatever caused their aggression.
- Never be patronizing or treat them with anything but respect. Remember, they're still adults with feelings and rights."[26] From Vantage Point Consulting, "De-escalation and Calming Techniques for Dementia Sufferers."

For the complete list and more information visit: https://vantagepointc.com/de-escalation-and-calming-techniques-for-dementia-sufferers/

I discovered my father's physician reviewed the basics of elder law with him and Marie on August 7, 2015, to ensure he had the proper documents for financial and medical decisions in place. By this time, my father had his directives completed for two years. However, the physician didn't confirm my father had them or identify his daughter as his healthcare proxy and power of attorney in his medical chart. If Marie had disclosed this information to my father's physician, it would have been documented in his report.

Your third layer of security

- I strongly suggest the healthcare proxy be invoked when a diagnosis is made. The healthcare advocate is permitted to receive all medical information and to make all decisions related to the person's medical treatment.
- I recommend healthcare advocates attend all appointments either in person, by Facetime or by Zoom.
- Relayed information from a caretaker or family member is not always complete or accurate. In my case, Marie intentionally omitted my father's healthcare and financial decisions to the Alzheimer's physicians.

My husband and I planned a high school graduation party for Danny, my stepson, at our house the same summer. My father and Marie came and stayed over for the weekend. It was quite a crowd, and many remembered my father from other parties we had and from our wedding. They reintroduced themselves to him. Before Alzheimer's, my father had always been the one who brought a sense of lightness and fun to a party. He said yes to every get-together and gathering when he asked to come. It didn't matter whose party it was or how few people he knew, because within minutes he'd be in a conversation. His knowledge spanned a wide range of subjects, from current events to historical facts and stories not that well known.

He was the person who piqued your interest and held your attention, but it was his reassuring manner that set him apart. When someone felt uncomfortable, he could tell by their energy. He knew how to bring them out of their shell, and he made them feel at ease. He talked about himself, but he did it to find some common ground, not for bragging.

He was the one you talked about after the party was over, the guy who left a lasting impression. But Alzheimer's was now leaving its impression. There was shame that my father carried. It wasn't his fault he didn't remember. It wasn't within his control. He didn't want to stand out. But his disease was taking over his identity. He craved normalcy, not pity. He just wanted to fit in.

At the party, my father came over beside me with his head lowered and whispered, "What town am I from?"

I quietly answered him, and he returned to the circle of people. I knew this day would come. Regardless, it still caught me off guard. His body language showed his embarrassment, but he didn't remove himself from the party.

The circle had dispersed, and he sat alone at the firepit, gazing into the flames. I glanced at him as I walked over the lawn towards the deck to go into the kitchen. For a split second, time stalled. It was like slow motion, and at that moment I looked at my father and I knew he knew.

Alzheimer's was the bully. It didn't hide its cruel nature. It was the constant and ever-threatening presence that attached itself to my father. There was nothing he could do, say, or wear to regain the feeling of being seen as normal again.

My father didn't want to be isolated. He loved being around his family and friends. The world was moving forward, and he didn't want to be left behind. My father said *yes* to life. If I was starting over this period of my father's life with him, I'd have encouraged him to come out and tell people who were close to him early on. I would have told him there is every reason to hold your head high.

There is no embarrassment in sharing incomplete thoughts. Forgetting where you came from has no relevance to where you are now. What matters is you are here. There is no shame in living.

LESSONS LEARNED

I've heard many people describe what it was like when they disclosed their cancer diagnosis. Some relationships turned awkward. It's not intentional but sometimes, good friends and even family avoid the person who is terminally diagnosed altogether because they don't know what to say or how to act.

What would you say to a person who told you they had Alzheimer's?

Or if you were at a party or gathering, and you found yourself in a group with a person who had Alzheimer's?

How would you navigate a conversation when a person stops speaking because they forgot the rest of their thought?

How would you react during an extended pause after you ask a person where they are from or where they live?

I'll tell you the answer. It can be as simple as a hand resting on a shoulder. There's no need to fill up dead air with words. It is the feeling of acceptance that makes a person feel included and valued.

Although my father didn't know where he was most of the time or where he was going, Marie booked five cruises beginning in November, leaving from Florida. 2016 would be the last year he could travel, she said. It didn't matter that he couldn't pack his suitcase, keep track of his wallet, or passport, know how to coordinate his clothing or even know when to shower. Just running an errand with him came with twenty questions, mostly one question repeated twenty times.

I called one day. They were between cruises, just getting home from one and packing for the next. I later found out in a conversation with Marie that these dream destinations were on her bucket list.

Marie said, "The Viking cruise was the ultimate."

She said, "They pampered us from the moment we boarded. They made each guest feel like royalty. I loved it. It's the best cruise I've ever been on!"

Marie showed Mark and me pictures of the other cruises. She described the shows at night and mentioned my father went to the restroom and got lost on the way back to her. She spoke of it as though it were an oops. Marie lowered her head and hunched her shoulders forward, then half smiled as she turned toward me. She laughed a little and said, "I should have gone with him."

I didn't bring it up in the conversation with her, but as a kid, I remember the feeling of being lost. It's scary and the fear and panic he must have felt, I can't imagine. Alzheimer's had changed my father's life in such a way that traveling caused more stress and frustration than joy and excitement. But regardless of how Alzheimer's made my father feel and the levels of anxiety and agitation it caused, it didn't prevent Marie from squeezing in every European destination and excursion she longed to see and experience.

I had mixed feelings before I understood why Marie had scheduled back-to-back trips. On the one hand, they were making trips of a lifetime. But five cruises? I thought if my father could enjoy traveling, it would be great. But this wasn't about taking leisurely laid-back trips, this was about checking off a list and completing it in a time frame that would make a normal person's head spin.

LESSONS LEARNED

"Sundowning can get worse when a person with dementia is sleep deprived. Theories of certain triggers that can make sundowning worse, including over-stimulation from a busy day."[27] From Cleveland Clinic, "Sundown Syndrome: Causes, Treatment & Symptoms."

Almost everyone would agree with me. The person's comfort level takes priority over following an itinerary and checking off a bucket list. If you want to fulfill a long-time dream destination trip, I advise a slower pace and scheduling daily rest periods. If excursions and sightseeing are a must, think about bringing along a family member who will enjoy staying with the person and doing more relaxing activities, while the other is out and about.

Chapter 11
The Opposition

Alzheimer's had sentenced my father, and it held him captive with no chance of a cure. Doctors couldn't revive the brain cells that had died, and I couldn't breathe new life into the ones that were dying. Alzheimer's had reinforced my helplessness.

2017 marked four years since his official diagnosis. According to the stages of the disease, the preclinical stage had probably begun years and possibly decades before. My father suffered from moderate to severe difficulty with recall. And at seventy-eight years old, his brain showed considerable atrophy.

I watched my father's physical appearance morph almost in unison with his mental decline. His once straight-as-an-arrow frame bent and leaned a little to the left. My father's gait stiffened as his tendons and ligaments lost their elasticity, and the muscles in his legs and hips tightened. The circulation within his body slowed, and one of his wrists and both ankles swelled periodically. But it was his eyes. They changed shape and became more rounded. There was a hollowness to them. Alzheimer's had manifested an emptiness in his eyes that I can only describe as a haunting vacancy.

My father didn't read the newspaper like he used to. Obituaries, headlines, and the sports page didn't spark any discussion, and I noticed how quickly he turned the pages. He looked like a child flipping through the pages of a book with no comprehension of the words written on the page. What used to take him about an hour to go through, now only took a couple of minutes.

On April 3, 2017, my father was diagnosed with stage 3b lung cancer, at the West Palm Beach VA Medical Center, while in Florida for the winter. On his medical record dated April 20, 2017, the oncology doctor noted that his son and daughter (me) were not aware of their father's cancer diagnosis. The oncology doctor also mentioned my father fully understood the healthcare proxy presented to him. My father named Marie as his advocate and signed it. This document became binding even though he forgot what he signed, the second after writing his name.

It was late afternoon on a Thursday. I was driving home from the Healing Garden after my workday when my phone rang. My father had trouble hearing and the spotty mobile reception on the back roads made it impossible to talk without having the call drop. As I pulled over onto a side street, I heard my father clear his throat. Marie was in the background.

My father said, "Hi, Jacqueline, it's Dad. I've got something to tell you. It's bad. I've got cancer."

"What kind, Dad? What's the prognosis?"

Marie filled in the rest because he couldn't remember.

Maries said, "It's stage 3b lung cancer. It's not operable but they can treat it and shrink the tumor. We have the appointments set up for chemo and radiation throughout the summer."

If my father had been clear-minded, he'd have called right away. He would have come home. However, Marie went forward with a treatment plan that was against my father's original healthcare proxy. And she waited until the second week of May, over three weeks after his diagnosis to tell me and my brother.

I went home and talked with Mark about planning a trip to Florida. In the meantime, my brother planned on booking a flight right away to see him. My father had a policy, at home, and in Florida, that his door was always open, and we were always welcome. Marie seemed to share his openness until now. Marie didn't want my brother and me to come to Florida together. She wanted to split our visits up. This came out of left field. Granted, she may have wanted some privacy, to digest the news, but it didn't seem that way. It felt rather odd because my brother and I had never been told not to visit together. It was out of character for Marie.

My brother arrived in Florida a couple of weeks before me. When he was in the kitchen, he saw a healthcare proxy naming Marie as my father's advocate. He sent a picture of it and texted: *"Aren't you dad's healthcare proxy?"*

I texted back, *yes*, and when I saw the VA Hospital header on the proxy that named Marie as his advocate, I wanted to know why. Yes, it would have been his right to make another proxy if a physician believed he could understand the document, but it was highly doubtful. I noticed Marie's cell phone number listed on his healthcare proxy. Then I noticed his initials and signature appeared shaky, and the answers in the boxes were checked off as *not sure*. This looked nothing like the specific terms and conditions stated in the healthcare proxy he made four years previously in 2013.

> The VA proxy:
> *If I am unconscious, in a coma, or a vegetative state and there is little to no chance of recovery.* My father initialed the box: *I'm not sure. It would depend on the circumstances.*
> *If I have permanent, severe brain damage that makes me unable to recognize my family or friends (for example, severe dementia).* He initialed again: *I'm not sure. It would depend on the circumstances.*

In seven out of seven questions, he initialed the same box *I'm not sure. It would depend on the circumstances.* With the other two choices being. *Yes. I would want life-sustaining treatments* and *No. I would not want life-sustaining treatments.*

My father's living will, signed on October 10, 2013, stated that:

> *I John J Sullivan willfully and voluntarily make known my desire that my dying not be artificially prolonged if:*
> *JJS. I have a terminal condition.*
> *JJS. I have an end-stage condition or,*
> *JJS. I am in a persistent vegetative state.*
> *And if there is no reasonable medical probability of my recovery from such a condition, I direct that*

> *life-prolonging procedures be withheld or withdrawn when the application of such procedures would serve only to prolong artificially the process of dying, and that I be permitted to die naturally with only the administration or the performance of any medical procedure deemed necessary to provide me with comfort care or to alleviate pain.*
>
> *It is my intention that this declaration be honored by my family and physician as the final expression of my legal right to refuse medical or surgical treatment or admission into a healthcare facility.*

My brother John and I knew what my father wanted. This new healthcare proxy didn't make sense. I asked my brother to speak to Marie and ask her when we could all talk. The next day, my brother called me and asked Marie while we were all on the line.

John said, "Marie, why did Dad make a healthcare proxy naming you when he has one? Jacqueline is Dad's healthcare proxy."

Marie said, "It was a mistake. I'm sorry. I feel awful. I didn't know your father named her."

I knew she was with my father when he drew up all his advanced directives two months after their wedding. His assets and medical decisions were legally defined and legally separated from Marie's. My father's documents were detailed, signed, and stamped. And even though I knew the facts Marie convinced me that maybe she did make a mistake.

I said, "Marie, we are asking you to come home. My father would want to be home with us. We want to be there for him and both of you. Mark feels the same."

Mark said, "Marie, the three of them are so close. This is going to be a lot and you may not realize it, but you are going to need help and support."

Marie said, "I'll think about it, Mark."

Marie had to be grieving. I tried to look at the situation from where she was, but I wanted her to understand how we felt. My brother and I made our case, and my husband reiterated how close we were. We were thankful, and we told her we appreciated her and the care she took of my father.

I said, "I can make the calls to transfer his treatment to Falmouth Hospital. Whatever you need, we can help. We can bring Dad to appointments to give you a break. This is a lot for one person to handle."

We called the next day, and she agreed, but she wanted to stay in Florida through his first round of chemo. She compromised, and we agreed immediately.

They came back in July to continue treatment. Mark and I met my brother John, Marie, and my father at the oncologist's initial meeting. While walking down the hallway, the secretary stopped the doctor, in front of me, to give him a copy of my father's living will and healthcare proxy. My father and Marie were already in his office waiting for him.

I said, "Excuse me, doctor. Can I speak to you without my father?"

He said, "Yes. We can go into the conference room."

My brother and husband were with me when the doctor asked me to explain my concerns.

I said, "In my father's living will, he stated that he would not want treatment if he had a terminal disease."

The doctor said, "Living wills in Massachusetts are invalid and have little to no bearing on treatment decisions."

That was news to me.

I asked, "How long will he have with treatment? And without treatment, how long?"

The doctor said, "Two years with and a few months without."

The doctor looked at me, my brother, and my husband.

He said, "Why wouldn't you treat him?"

Then he excused himself. I did not want my father to die. This decision not to prolong my father's life if he had a terminal diagnosis, with no chance of recovery, came from my father. He now had two life-threatening diseases, one of which would send him into the vegetative state he never wanted to live in.

In 2017, my father had increasingly poor judgment, deepening confusion and even greater memory loss. The doctor called me into the office after he examined my father. I sat next to him with Marie on his opposite side. As I spoke to the doctor about my father, he corrected me.

He said, "Your father is here. Talk to him."

I said, "Dad, you have Alzheimer's and lung cancer," then I choked on my words, "If you continue cancer treatment, your Alzheimer's is still going to get worse, and it is going to be a slower way to die. You have always told me if your brain died and there was no chance of recovery, you would rather die than be kept alive."

His memory of the decisions he made in his living will were gone. I knew it when he looked at me.

My father said, "I don't care, whatever, it doesn't matter to me."

My father didn't remember he had Alzheimer's or lung cancer and when I heard his reply, I felt like I was going to be sick. I hated this. I was more unsure of what to do. And I went against my gut and continued with treatment.

The doctors supported Marie and her decision to move forward with the cancer treatments. Marie set into motion medical treatment that went against my father's wishes. Once he signed another healthcare proxy in Florida, naming Marie, her opinions on what my father's treatment should be, became the care he received. Her beliefs and opinions on what my father's care should be snowballed and carried over into Massachusetts.

LESSONS LEARNED

There's a thin line between a physician's legal duty and refusal to honor a patient's medical decisions. A family member's opinions and beliefs can influence the physician's decisions over the patient's treatment.

"Health care providers have a duty to provide care. Their values, however, can sometimes conflict with these duties. Is it acceptable to deny a patient care if it goes against the provider's morals, ethics, or religious beliefs? That is when conscientious objection comes into play. A conscientious objection in medicine is the refusal to provide the requested treatment due to the provider's moral convictions. Physicians are not obligated to adhere to the decisions of a healthcare proxy when their religious beliefs and ethical or moral opinions differ."[28] From the Yale School of Medicine, When Personal and Professional Morals Clash: Conscientious Objection in Medicine, by Crystal Gwizdala.

The Opposition

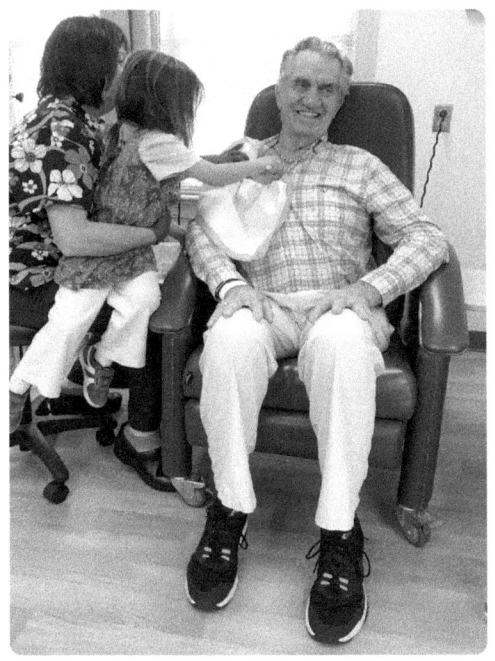

John's daughter Beverly and her grandfather John (Jack) Sullivan at chemotherapy on October 5, 2017.
Photo by John Sullivan, author's brother, with permission.

My brother John, and my niece Beverly, who was four at the time, never missed going on the days of my father's chemotherapy infusion. My husband went with my father when I was working. After one month, I needed reaffirmation that we were doing the right thing. In August, I emailed my father's radiologist and asked him to clarify the treatment and the prognosis.

-Original Message-----
From Jacqueline Sullivan
Sent: Friday, August 11, 2017, 8:02 am
To: C-- MD,
Subject: J Sullivan
I have a couple of questions. My family and I met you on Tues. My dad is 78 years old with Alzheimer's and stage 3b lung cancer.

I am not clear on what Dr. Max, the Alzheimer's physician, had said. You had mentioned a year out my dad could be worse or several months out, depending on how the disease progressed. I have a call into him also to clarify. It's difficult to ask questions when my dad is there.

> *Dr. G. had mentioned radiation, not chemo and radiation together.*
> *Why both together?*
> *What if he just had the radiation and not chemo again?*
> *I understand that stage 3b cancer usually returns. If the tumor does go away how much time before it returns?*
> *If he just had the radiation, where would he be in terms of survival time?*
> *If it is easier to talk, you can reach me at _____ If I don't answer, can you please leave a time when it's best to call you back?*
> *Thank you so much,*
> *I appreciate it.*
> *Jacqueline Sullivan Wyco*

The radiologist replied to me with the email he sent to my father's Alzheimer's physician, Dr. Max.

> *On Aug 11, 2017, at 10:07 am,*
> *The radiologist stated, My question to Dr. Max was whether Alzheimer's was an immediate threat to his life. He classifies it as mild to moderate and he expects this would not be life threatening for at least several years. Cancer is an imminent threat within months if no further treatment is given.*
> *The combination of chemo and radiation is far more effective than radiation alone in a situation like this and does give us the potential to eradicate this, which I do not think would be reasonable with radiation alone. The chemo involved here is single and a much lower dose than he received before, and the oncology doctor supports this. When he met with you, he wasn't sure if radiation was feasible. Since meeting with you, I obtained his prior PET scan,*

which I have attached with a comparison to his new scan. I think radiation is very reasonable given this excellent response. More importantly, his physical condition is very good. His Alzheimer's might become life-threatening within the next several years, but the possibility of rapidly growing lung cancer concerns me, as this can be very symptomatic if it grows locally, makes his breathing very difficult, and creates a very miserable existence.

Alzheimer's had abolished my father's independence. Managing irritability, agitation, anxiety, and restlessness had risen to the top of the daily to-do list. He was incapable of living on his own. He could not make a simple piece of toast or a cup of tea. His tendency to fall increased. Wounds took longer to heal, like the six-inch long gash along his shin from a fall he took in the shower. Losing his phone had become a daily occurrence. If there was an emergency, or he became lost, and he had to use another phone, he wouldn't know how to use it or know who to call. But the doctors felt "More importantly, his physical condition was very good. And his Alzheimer's **might** become life-threatening within the next several years."

My father was living in a state of continuous mental and physical decline, with no reasonable medical probability of recovery. But the doctors and Marie wanted to treat lung cancer so my father could live longer, and in doing so, he would die more slowly.

Life is a gift, but this was not the gift of life my father wanted or chose. The doctors did not consider that it was my father's right to refuse treatment that would extend his life if he were terminal with no chance of a cure. This granted consent to the disease that had already seized the very essence of what it meant for my father to live a full and happy life.

◇◇◇

On a day off, I visited my father and Marie on the Cape. He was in bed when I arrived. I sat with Marie at the kitchen table while she made a pot of coffee. My father was a hugger and that didn't change during his Alzheimer's. When he got up in the morning, he hugged us. When he went to bed, he hugged and kissed us on the cheek goodnight, and the same when we said hello or goodbye. And Marie did too since we met her. But on this day, she acted differently. She was at the counter pouring her coffee when my father came downstairs and hugged her good morning. After she finished fixing her coffee, she sat at the table with me while my father grabbed his.

Marie said to me, "I'm not a touchy-feely person."

This was one of those confusing moments. She hugged my father and returned our hugs for 19 years. I didn't understand where that came from. Coincidently, a week or so prior, my brother called me to talk about my father's decline before his yearly visit with the Alzheimer's physician. He said he noticed a change in Marie.

He said, "She's different and it happened once Dad gave her the ring. Shouldn't you be taking care of Dad's finances?"

Marie grew more controlling throughout my father's decline. I thought it was because of his disease, and I still didn't relate her control to anything malicious. It was time I talked with her about invoking my father's power of attorney and taking over his finances like he set up for me to do. But I knew from experience that it may not go over well.

On the day of my father's appointment, Mark and I met my father and Marie, at the Alzheimer's office, on the south shore, close to the Cape. When my father was called into the doctor's office, I approached the subject of finances with Marie.

I said, "Marie, I think it's time I take over my father's finances."

Her body tightened and grew rigid. Her jaw clenched as she tightly held a magazine open on her lap. She didn't want to have this conversation, and her body language said it all. She planted both feet flat on the ground and pushed her knees tightly together.

She said, "You're interfering in my marriage."

She returned to her magazine. I explained again that this was what my father wanted, and it was what he set up for me to do.

This time, she raised her head abruptly. In a more forceful tone, she said, "I'll think about it."

There was another person in the waiting room. In public wasn't the best place to have this conversation. But I'm glad I didn't do this in private. I didn't let Marie's avoidance deter me.

I said, "No, Marie, it's happening."

And I left it at that.

We were called into the office and Marie's first question to the doctor was about my father's finances.

Marie said, "Jack's daughter wants to take over her father's finances. What is your opinion?"

The Alzheimer's doctor said, "It's actually past the time that power of attorney should have been taking care of his finances and if I were called to testify in court, it's what I would say."

Marie's entire demeanor softened in the doctor's presence. She retreated and listened to him. The doctor dictated the notes of our meeting into his computer microphone while we were there.

I said, "I'll call you, Marie, to set up a day to pick up and go over my father's records."

The day I went to the Cape, Marie answered the door. She looked like she had been up for quite some time. It was still early, about 10 am. She had makeup on and wore a heather grey long skirt with a yoga top that matched with a print. She was always put together.

She smiled and said, "I have everything ready for you. Your father's file case is on the kitchen table. I can show you what's in it."

She asked, "Would you like coffee or water?"

I said, "Thank you, sure, I'll have water, thank you."

Marie seemed to have a complete turnaround in attitude.

She said, "Oh, this will work out fine."

I didn't stay long, and it went better than expected.

My brother informed me a week later that Marie had offered to go to the bank with him to put his name on the accounts. I was the power of attorney, and my brother was the alternate.

Marie was keeping me at arm's length, something she hadn't done before. I met my brother at my father's home. My father and Marie drove separately to the bank. I went in my vehicle and my brother took his. Marie came in with us and sat in a chair in the open lobby. I saw her off to the side in the corner of my eye. She bounced her leg and tried not to stare as I added my name to my father's accounts.

LESSONS LEARNED

Your fourth layer of security is going to work to prevent financial loss.

I advise the person with power of attorney to take 5 steps once a diagnosis is made:

1. Speak to the person's physician and get invoked ASAP. This will create an overlap in security.
2. Add name, with the title of power of attorney, to financial accounts
3. Change billing address to power of attorney and take over bills immediately.
4. For online accounts, change usernames, and passwords. Monitor accounts monthly.
5. Create transparency by keeping a ledger. At the end of each month, forward it to other advocates and close family members.

After two months of radiation, my father developed side effects. The radiation-induced red rash caused itching, oozing, and a burning sensation. He developed mouth sores, a sore throat, brain fog, loss of concentration, nausea, and intermittent diarrhea.

The energy reserves in my father's body went to repair the damage radiation and chemo caused, leaving him with fatigue that worsened as the treatments progressed. For every side effect, there was a new medication to add. They helped, but his agitation and confusion related to Alzheimer's intensified. My father had aggressive lung cancer, and the treatments combined with where he was in Alzheimer's made his life miserable. He was suffering and in pain.

On October 8, 2017, I emailed my father's radiologist and explained that my father was having adverse effects from the treatment, and on the weekend, his symptoms took a turn for the worse.

> *Hi Dr.,*
> *This weekend my father's Alzheimer's took a turn for the worse. After discussions with my family and Dr.Max, we have decided to stop all treatment. Effective immediately. I am aware that he has 6 treatments left.*
> *This discussion is based on what my father, in his sound mind, would want. He is on so many medications and now having events of severe anger, confusion, and extreme fatigue. This is not quality of life and a tortuous way to live.*
>
> *Thank you,*
> *Jacqueline Sullivan Wyco*

His radiologist responded that although he had developed some skin toxicity from the treatment which will resolve, he asked if it would be okay to follow up with him relatively soon to monitor his side effects.

In the meantime, I had questions for my father's new oncologist, who replaced his previous doctor who retired. I couldn't speak with her directly that day, so the secretary in the office suggested I contact his radiologist to answer my questions regarding his care. I emailed the radiologist on Oct. 18, 2017, and confirmed that we had a follow-up appointment with him, as he suggested, but I did not want to ask in front of my father.

I said, "Looking ahead, as far as pain management, should I contact and set up palliative care or hospice so someone can see him weekly to assess how he is doing? Or would he need scans first before that is determined?"

The goal of palliative care is symptom management, and it could have been provided in my father's home. I asked the radiologist about beginning palliative care because I wanted his symptoms to be managed before they grew out of control. However, the radiologist didn't feel palliative care or hospice was necessary at this time.

Fear Knocked — Jacqueline Sullivan Wyco

We all met at the hospital on the day of his follow-up oncology appointment. My brother John, my husband Mark, my niece Beverly, myself, Marie, and my father sat together in the radiologist's office. The doctor reviewed his latest scans with us, assessed his skin, and then addressed Marie. She asked him a question before our appointment that day and we weren't aware of it until the doctor answered her.

The radiologist said, "Dr. Max, the Alzheimer's physician, and I have discussed, and we agree that there is no reason why you and your husband cannot return to Florida for the winter."

My brother and I both adjusted ourselves in our seats. It was the first time either of us had heard about Marie's plan to go back to Florida on November 8, 2017, for the winter. My brother and I were hesitant. He had been through so much. We didn't want him to go, yet we wanted him to live his life and be happy for however much or little time he had left.

The radiologist said, "You can make an appointment to remove his port." The port allowed needle-free blood drawings and chemotherapy treatments. It was implanted in a vein in his upper chest.

Marie asked, "Could we have the port removed in Florida?"

The radiologist said, "Yes. that would be fine."

Marie said, "I'll make the appointment when we get to Florida." Marie reassured me when we sat together in the hallway after our meeting to get a coffee for my father.

Marie said, "If your father gets worse, we'll come home early."

I planned to fly down every six weeks to check on him. My husband came with me for the first visit, a week before Christmas. My father seemed okay. During our stay, I asked Marie about my father's friend. "Marie, how's Murray?"

She said, "We don't talk to him anymore."

I couldn't believe it. Murray and my father were friends for forty-plus years. He lived downstairs on the first floor of their condo building in Florida. He moved there after my father called him to let him know that the unit had gone up for sale. He loved Murray and his wife. They were great, great friends.

Originally, Marie got along well with them: they became friends. But after Murray's wife died and after my father's condition worsened, suddenly there was a rift. When I asked my father what happened, he just scowled. Marie told me two things. One, she didn't know why my father felt that way. Two, she was mad at Murray because he had walked into their condo without any warning.

Marie said, "He didn't knock and walked in unannounced. I wasn't dressed. I had just gotten out of the shower."

Marie said, "Murray let himself in before. It's not the first time. He always walks right in."

My father's relationship with Murray had been solid. I didn't see how their relationship could break down from walking in a door without knocking. I wondered why Marie didn't lock the door, so Murray would have to knock before entering. Then the problem would have been solved.

Yes, my father had Alzheimer's, and his disease could have made up a fight in his mind, but what about Marie? She seemed to reinforce the rift when she could have easily mended their friendship by reminding my father of their history.

Their partnership in the fire department went beyond camaraderie. They had a bond. My father told the story periodically through the years. Marie heard it and knew how tight they were.

On a fire scene, Murray and my father were opening a roof when they got trapped on a widow's walk. The ceilings were collapsing as the fire moved up through the first, second, and third floors. The roof turned spongy. It was going next, and so were they if they didn't get off. But the smoke turned black and got thicker as the fire roared out of control. It was impossible to see the ladder to climb down.

Calmly, they both resigned themselves to the fact they were going to die. Just then, a gust of wind opened a path to where they saw the tip of the ladder. He called it the stick. They ran and made one dive. A split second longer and they wouldn't have made it. In recent years, Murray helped my father through some tough times. In years prior, my father had been there for him.

It wasn't clear then, but a pattern was evolving behind the separation and division of friendships my father shared, especially of those who knew him well. And I didn't know why.

About six weeks later, in February 2018, I flew to Florida, with my brother. Mostly, we hung out with my father. In the evening, we watched TV. One night I went to bed early, and my brother stayed up with Marie and my father. As I closed the bedroom door, I heard Marie ask my brother. *What did your sister do with all the money?* He told her he didn't know.

Before I took over my father's finances, Marie told me they spent a lot of money. I was aware of their lifestyle. They frequently dined out and went on cruises and trips. They enjoyed themselves. But even though their finances were separate, she showed great concern about the whereabouts of his money.

I asked my father's financial advisor for advice. To safeguard his accounts, I opened a new account, linked it to my father's checking and savings accounts, and added my brother as an owner to the account. I kept enough money in his checking account for the automatic withdrawal bills and for the cash that Marie withdrew twice a week. I put the overflow into the new account.

The next day, we all sat at the pool for a while. My father loved the ocean, the sun, and the fresh air. That was his medicine, even during his Alzheimer's. We sat at a table near the canal, watched boats go by, and just enjoyed being outside. My brother went with my father to the restroom so he could find his way back to our table.

Marie made small talk while they were gone. She mentioned selling their Cape house. I was thinking, *How? Because it's in an irrevocable trust, why would she want to sell the condo on the Cape?* The plan was always for my father to be back home in Massachusetts with our family. When my father returned to the table, he looked at me funny.

He said, "And who are you?"

My father wasn't joking. Marie was sitting next to me on my left. I couldn't see her when I answered my father.

I said, "Dad, I'm Jacqueline, your daughter."

I looked at my brother and thought, *my god*.

Marie shifted gears and said to my father, "If you could live on the Cape or Florida, what would you choose?"

He looked dazed. Then he looked straight at Marie. First, he stuttered a bit, as if unsure of what to say.

He said, "Ca...pe?"

Then he paused as if he was solving a puzzle. He pointed his finger down towards the table and shook his head up and down.

He said, "Cape Cod."

Then shook his head, "Oh. No. Here? In Florida?"

I wasn't looking at Marie. It would be much later before I realized she had prompted him.

I called the Alzheimer's physician when I got home and left a message about my father and the progression of the disease.

I said, "My father doesn't know where he is in his own house. He didn't remember I was his daughter. He's looking for his mother, who isn't alive, and his agitation is increasing. What should I do and where should he be?"

I was at work when he returned my call. His advice to me was that my father should be in hospice, which meant he had six months or fewer to live, and he should be where he was going to die. I told the doctor he was in Florida and that because of the difficulty I had with Marie, I asked if he could reach out to her.

The Alzheimer's physician said, "No, I don't get involved in family matters."

I called Marie after I got home. Mark was there, and I had my phone on speaker. I told her exactly what the doctor said, then she shouted to my father. "Jack, they all think you're going to die, and they want you to go home."

My father didn't remember he had Alzheimer's, and this not only confused him, but it also made him angry.

He said, "Who thinks I'm going to die?"

Marie said, "Jacqueline, John, and Mark. They all think you're going to die."

My father yelled in the background. "TELL THEM TO LEAVE US ALONE!"

Marie said, "I'll think about it. I have things to do. I have appointments. Physical therapy. An eye doctor's appointment. And a life!"

Mark said, "Marie, can you please call us back and talk in private, without Jack in the room?"

Days went by with no response, no text, no call.

I couldn't wait any longer. I stopped by the firehouse, to see Mark at work.

I said, "Can you please try texting Marie? Maybe she'll respond to you."

Marie texted him back and told us what day we could talk. We reminded her that my father should not be in the room where he could hear our conversation.

Mark said, "Marie, you can't talk about Alzheimer's with Jack in the room because he doesn't remember he has Alzheimer's. He doesn't understand. It will only agitate him."

The day came, and I was nervous. This had to go well. I had to keep my composure, and I asked Mark to speak first. He had a gentle way of smoothing out a disagreement, and Marie liked him.

On the speaker, my husband went through again what the Alzheimer's physician said.

He said, "Jack needs to be home and where he is going to die. This is not Jacqueline's opinion. It's what the doctor said. Why don't you call him and talk with him?"

Marie got ticked off.

She said, "I will!"

She then turned the focus to herself.

She said, "I have appointments, an art project, an art show at the end of the month."

I drew NO on a piece of paper at the kitchen table and circled it multiple times as I shook my head no and mouthed *come home*. I tried to keep out of it and let Mark handle it. But I stayed quiet as long as I could. When Marie went on about her art class, I lost it.

I said, "Marie, my father is dying. He needs to be in hospice and if we wait too long, we may not get him home!"

I was beside myself. My father's end-of-life decisions were not Marie's priority, and, in her words, "It's not what I want."

I said, "This isn't about you, Marie!"

She flat-out refused again.

She said, "I'm not coming home. I don't care what the doctor said. I'm staying."

I said, "Okay. Marie, I'm coming down and I'm bringing my father and his car home."

She said, "Go ahead, come and get him, take him to your house."

She dared me. This wasn't your textbook definition of grief.

LESSONS LEARNED

- I urge you to include a social worker in your care team from day one.
- Routine meetings are an opportunity to resolve issues among family members and advocates.
- Separate and divide is a tactic used by manipulators to gain power and control over a person. Ask questions about a sudden move, rifts or estrangements with family.
- Communication creates transparency and can eliminate power grabs.
- The documentation along the stages of the disease will help protect your loved one and their decisions if ever they become the subject of a court case.

"Social workers are frequently called to testify as experts in courts of law on a variety of subjects. Courts rely on information offered in evidence as the basis for decisions rendered, and oral testimony by witnesses is often the major source of evidence provided at a trial. This law note discusses the role of social workers as expert witnesses and reviews case law confirming their role as experts in a variety of legal settings."[29] From the National Association of Social Workers.

Chapter 12
The Ultimatum

The Alzheimer's doctor's six-month timeline panicked me. I wanted to bring my father home so he could die, surrounded by his family. And this enraged Marie. It didn't concern her the way I thought it would.

My father had permitted me to move him as his power of attorney. Theoretically, I had the legal right to go to Florida and bring him home after his primary care physician signed the letter of incapacitation, giving me the authority as his advocate. Mark and I were still in the kitchen after we hung up with Marie in Florida.

"Mark, I'm going to Florida and bringing my father home."

Mark said, "You can't just rip him out of there. He's attached to Marie."

I needed a solution, one that wouldn't cause my father any unnecessary added stress and one that would defuse Marie.

I said, "Mark, what about your parents' attorney? Do you have his number?"

I called the attorney and asked his opinion on my situation and guardianship. He told me, I already had power of attorney. I didn't need guardianship to bring my father home. I was more confused than ever. The attorney in Florida made it sound like I needed guardianship. In the meantime, my brother was working on getting an appointment with another attorney, referred to us by a friend, to review my father's directives. We wanted to understand the terms and conditions my father spelled out in his directives. Until our meeting, it appeared the best option was to bring my father home with Marie. That meant I needed to come up with a compromise to which she would agree.

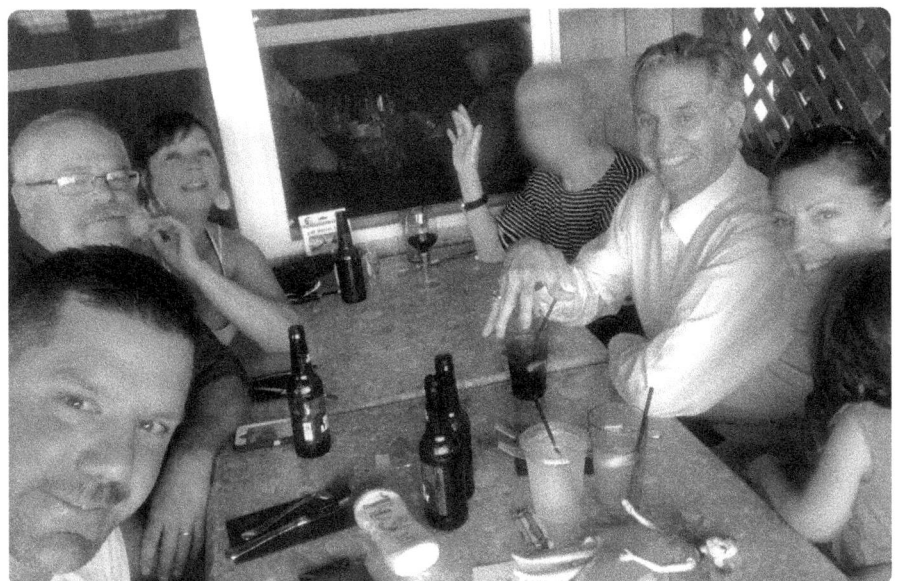

August 27, 2017 Birthday Lunch For Marie: Left John, Jacqueline's brother, behind him Mark Wyco, Jacqueline's husband next, author, Jacqueline. Front right Beverly, Karen Sullivan John's wife, next John Sullivan, back right Marie. *Photo taken by John Sullivan, printed with permission by John and Karen Sullivan, and Mark Wyco.*

I called Marie back after a couple of hours and explained that I could fly down and stay with them until the end of the month, after her art show. I knew she wasn't thrilled, but she agreed to it.

I didn't have the official authority yet to make healthcare decisions on my father's behalf. So, next, I called my father's primary care doctor on the Cape to explain my father's symptoms. And on March 7, 2018, the Invocation of Healthcare Surrogate, that named me, went into place. I was now in control of all my father's safety, medical, financial, and legal matters. His primary care physician signed it. To provide further help, the physician added a clinical patient advocate to contact.

When I went to Florida, I needed to let go of what happened with Marie. My father loved and trusted her, and he picked up on the energy of those around him. The last thing he needed was to feel tension. On my way from the airport to the condo, I texted Marie that I was on the way. She texted back, *come in, the door is unlocked.* When I arrived, they were in the living room watching the local nightly news. I walked over to my father and kissed him on the cheek, then over to

Marie to do the same, but she turned away. From the moment I came in, Marie wanted me to leave. I was in the guest room, getting ready for bed, when I heard Marie shouting. I opened my door to find out what was going on.

Marie said, "She's interfering in our relationship. I want her gone! She's an intruder. Jacqueline and John are controlling you. You will never come back to Florida because they don't want you to."

Marie used the distortion in my father's brain to manipulate him. She gave him an ultimatum. She said, "You need to tell her to leave. If you don't, I'll leave you!"

My father grew tormented. He was so confused and upset. I saw it on his face.

He said, "You'll leave me?"

Marie said, "Yup."

I said, "What's going on?"

Marie kept going. It was so bad I called home to Mark and had him listen while I tried to get her to stop badgering my father.

I said, "Marie, please stop. Why are you doing this?"

Marie's behavior threw me off. I didn't know what to do. All I wanted was for her to stop. She finally calmed down and I returned to my room. But the tensions worsened as the days went on. Marie walked by me as if I weren't there. She spoke to my father to relay information to me and then convinced him I caused the tensions between her and me.

Marie tried to get me to leave by making me as uncomfortable as possible. The silent treatment began on my arrival. But Marie told my father I was silently punishing her. The next morning, my father came over to me as I sat having my coffee in the kitchen while Marie dressed and finished her makeup in their bedroom.

My father said, "Marie's a good person. Can't you try to get along with her and talk to her? I love you both."

He didn't understand what was happening, nor did I. But I realized quickly that Marie was fighting to stay in Florida permanently with my father. Marie and I never argued in all the years I had known her. Not so much as a tiff. It was just last summer that my family and I surprised Marie for her birthday. We met her and my father in Wellfleet at The Bookstore Restaurant across from the beach. She thought we were just meeting for lunch, but we surprised her for her birthday. My brother, his wife, and my niece, together with myself and Mark, celebrated with small gifts and a dessert with a candle. We loved her. Marie even commented to my father what a nice family he had. But this was normal for us as a family. Over the years, Marie came to my house for the holidays, and all sorts of parties, including a Father's Day barbecue to which Mark and I invited her kids, their family, and in-laws. Often, we had gatherings for no other reason than just getting together. My brother and I both welcomed her into our homes and our family. Yet, since I arrived in Florida, she treated me as though I were an outcast.

In Florida, I wanted to spend time with my father, but in doing so, I also had to be with Marie. She never left his side or left me with him alone since I arrived at the condo. One afternoon, while watching TV with them, a commercial about receiving a check came on. It seemed to jog my father's memory.

My father asked, "Marie, didn't we just get a check?"

Her body stiffened as she had before in the Alzheimer's physician's office, and she stared straight ahead. She didn't look at me and she hesitated.

She said, "No."

Alzheimer's gave Marie leverage. As my father became more impaired, Marie grew more emboldened. In a twisted form of gaslighting, Marie turned my father's lucid moment into a memory that never happened. I didn't know who to believe. Marie took my father out for hours at a time. One morning she left, she took out the trash and put a fresh bag in the basket. I went to throw away something when I saw a piece of paper on top. I picked it up. The note was made out to Marie from the postwoman, Linda. *I will continue to hold Jack's mail.* Everyone in the condo community knew Linda. She was fond of my father. And with the heart she signed the note with, it appeared she cared about Marie. My father's mail was kept from me seeing it, on purpose. But why? I didn't know but I immediately put the note in my binder, into my backpack, and walked to the post office with my invoked healthcare proxy and power of attorney. There, I filled out paperwork to get my father's mail.

Fear Knocked — Jacqueline Sullivan Wyco

The note the author found from Linda, the postwoman, to Marie. *From the records collected by the author*

When Marie took my father out, I looked for clues to explain her behavior. While in the kitchen, I saw a calendar on the desk with oncology infusion appointments. I didn't question Marie because we had ended his treatment before he returned to Florida. I thought they were old appointments. However, I asked her about a confirmation letter I saw lying on the counter for a canceled appointment.

Marie said, "It was a follow-up appointment with the doctor and your father didn't need to go because he felt better."

I ripped it up and tossed it. That night, I had trouble sleeping. I needed to confirm the appointment I threw away. The next morning, I picked through the trash and put the pieces I had torn the appointment into in my backpack with some tape, and down to the clubhouse I went.

When I called the hospital and asked what the appointment was for, I was told it was for a social worker, not an appointment for a check-up. Marie never mentioned my father having a social worker and if he did, why did she feel the need to cover it up? I was sitting in the back of the clubhouse when Marie walked in. She didn't see me. A friend of theirs walked up to her and asked, "How's our Jack doing?"

Marie said, "He's doing well, and the tumor is shrinking."

It sounded as if he were still in treatment, but we had ended the treatment. My mind started working backward, and I wanted to know what the oncology appointments were that I saw earlier and dismissed.

I went back to the condo and waited until Marie left with my father before I called the hospital again. I identified myself as my father's daughter and his invoked power of attorney and healthcare proxy. They denied me the information. I called again, and they redirected me to the oncology department. I talked to the nurse, Dolly, and explained who I was, and she confirmed my father had two drug infusions on December 4, 2017. This was two months after we stopped cancer treatment on the Cape in Massachusetts.

There were two drugs listed and when I asked what drugs they were, I was told they were chemotherapy drugs. To be clear, I asked again. I couldn't believe what I was hearing. Chemo had caused my father such adverse side effects, so why did Marie go against my father's wishes and our agreement as a family? We ended chemo in October and my father's port was supposed to be taken out in Florida and it wasn't. Marie made an appointment, and my father received more chemo. Then she made the appointment for the port to be taken out before Mark and I visited them in Florida. Marie's sudden shift in behavior and my discoveries were clues. The fragments of information formed a narrative that didn't match Marie's chronicle of events. It was coming together, and I felt like everything I thought I knew just blew apart into a million pieces.

Marie and my father were still gone. I wanted to call Mark. But I didn't want to risk them overhearing my conversation if they came home. So, I walked out to the balcony down near the end unit in the corner behind the open stairwell. My voice trembled. When I started talking, I began sobbing uncontrollably. Mark couldn't understand me. I lost my breath while explaining what I had just found out. He helped me calm down.

Mark said, "Your father, right now, is okay. Focus on that."

I had to get it together. I didn't want Marie to get any hint of what I discovered because I needed to find out more.

That morning, I made fourteen calls to the VA Hospital in West Palm Beach. I tried to find out why my father had chemotherapy after we stopped treatment. When I got off the phone, I took an Uber to the hospital with my power of attorney and healthcare proxy/living will. The receptionist at the sign-in desk referred me to social services.

Fear Knocked — Jacqueline Sullivan Wyco

The social worker assigned to my father's case was standoffish even after I explained who I was and why I was there. I asked her to put my power of attorney, healthcare proxy, and the letter of incapacitation for my father in his file. I told her we stopped treatment before my father came back to Florida and we agreed as a family, but she didn't react like I expected.

The social worker remained distant and unconcerned when I showed her my father's original healthcare proxy/living will and the one he had filled out at their hospital on April 27, 2017. I pointed out the major differences between the two.

Then I laid out on her desk the evaluation by the Alzheimer's physician, which was dated before my father returned to Florida, and it revealed *severe cognitive impairment*. I placed their medical evaluation notes next to it, which repeatedly stated my father had been *cognitively aware and understood the course of treatment*. She became flustered when she couldn't explain it.

The social worker said, "I'm sorry, I need to call my supervisor."

I waited in the cubby hole-sized office for her supervisor. All the while the social worker avoided looking at me. When the manager arrived, I repeated my problem to her. But she couldn't explain it either. She told me she would look into it and get back to me.

I returned to the condo and kept looking. In a book, I found notes on long-term care facilities, and in another book, The 36 Hour Day, I found pages that were dog-eared with notes. I'd seen it on the kitchen counter in their Cape house. The more I looked, the more questions I had. The real estate business card clipped to the calendar and a wire transfer receipt in my father's handwriting told me that Marie had plans for the very near future.

I wanted to lay it all out for Marie, but I couldn't. There had to be more. I had to distance myself from her because when I asked Marie a question, she took it as a confrontation and became defensive. This would have made her more volatile than she already was. Marie had a plan and after finding the notes on long-term care facilities in her book, I knew I was at risk of losing him.

The Ultimatum

LESSONS LEARNED

My father loved, trusted, and depended on Marie. People with Alzheimer's are easily intimidated by those whom they trust and depend on. My father was fearful at the moment Marie threatened to leave him. I discovered, "Coercive control is the pattern of behavior or actions used by a perpetrator to frighten, threaten, oppress, and limit their victim. A perpetrator will work to isolate and intimidate their partner to the point where their partner's isolation from others and dependence on them gives them an immense feeling of power and control."[30] From Domestic Violence Network, "Coercive Control: Abuse Hidden in Plain Sight."

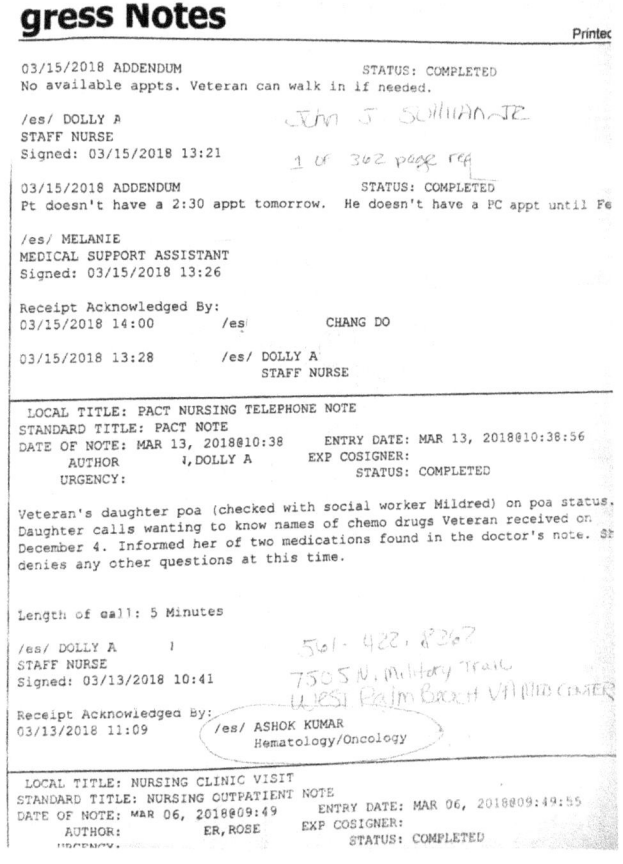

Jacqueline's father's medical records were obtained by her brother John at the VA Hospital in West Palm Beach, FL in the third week of March 2018. VA Hospital West Palm Beach notes stating the author had called asking what drugs her father received after treatment was stopped.
From the records collected by the author

Chapter 13
Optical Illusion

People believe what they see with their own eyes. Marie appeared to be the doting wife and caretaker. No one saw anything other than what Marie portrayed, except for me recently, and that was behind closed doors.

Marie said she wanted to go to Florida with my father after we ended cancer treatment to get out of the long winter in Massachusetts. And I believed her. The 1,500 miles between my father and my family shielded Marie's pursuit of guardianship. Marie was on a mission. She tried to remove me as my father's advocate legally. Breaking my relationship with my father would have strengthened her case against me.

I chased information and tried to find out what Marie did, but defending my father became a race where Marie had the overall advantage. For the month I stayed in Florida, I ran on fear and adrenalin. Marie blindsided me. I didn't know if I was acting quickly enough to protect my father and his assets. Depending on how long it took, it might be too late. My solution: Block the threat. Investigate later.

I didn't monitor any of my father's assets, including his IRA. I never asked Marie about the money she withdrew from his checking account or how she spent it. But the check my father mentioned stuck with me. There were few spaces in the condo complex where I talked in private. It was a tight-knit community. They all watched out for each other and news traveled like wildfire. My father's neighbors were friendly. They knew everything that went on there, from who had visitors, where they were from, and how long they were staying. And that included me.

I went down to the pool area early in the morning to make my calls. I sat with my back against a wall and kept my voice down. Many people genuinely cared about my father and Marie. There weren't too many people who didn't know them. They only knew me from what they heard about me. And depending on how they perceived me through Marie, only one needed to overhear me to send the news directly back to Marie. If she discovered I was engaged in protecting my father and his assets, she might have sped up whatever plans she already had in motion.

I called the three credit reporting agencies and explained my father was incapacitated by Alzheimer's and I was his invoked power of attorney. I asked for an investigation into the financial activity in his credit report. Specifically, if someone took any loans out and if any new credit cards were opened. However, before receiving any information, I needed to mail a hard copy of the power of attorney. Emailing documents wasn't permitted to speed up the process. Even with an existing threat, I had to wait until they processed the power of attorney before freezing his credit. Typically, it takes seven to ten business days to process from receiving it. To prevent access to his IRA, I prepared to move it laterally to another institution. They instructed me to print out a form to have it notarized and then mail it with my power of attorney. This, again, was going to take seven to ten business days. Every piece of information I accumulated, I kept secure in my backpack.

I tried to think and move quickly, and mentally it caught up to me. It was my birthday, and I had just hit a wall. I needed a breather. It was a nice day, so I walked to the community pool. I usually sat near the wall at the back, closer to the exit, where it was quieter. But the only chairs available at the peak time of day were sandwiched in the middle of the large crowd.

The two ladies, who sat one chair away from me, spoke feverishly back and forth. My ears perked when I heard my father's name, then Marie's. Then it came.

One said, "And how about that daughter? Marie said she's after all the money."

The two ladies leaned into each other, half whispering. They couldn't gossip fast enough. They were like piranhas in a feeding frenzy, and they kept going. As I listened, I wanted to say something. But I wasn't sure if I should. Of all things, I was reading a meditation book when I felt a supercharged rush of adrenaline. I took a deep breath and walked over to them.

I said, "Excuse me, I'm Jack's daughter and what you are saying isn't true."

Their jaws dropped open, and their faces froze as they leaned away from each other, back into their chairs.

I said, "You shouldn't be gossiping about something when you do not know what you are talking about. You don't know me, or my family, and you don't know what my father set up for me to do. I love my father, and I appreciate Marie caring for him, but that goes both ways. My father took very good care of her for years."

When I finished, they defended Marie.

Both said, "She is our friend."

I stood in front of them.

I said, "There are three sides to every story to which you heard only one."

The two ladies said, "We are very sorry. Your father is a very nice man."

I felt like I was on fire, and I walked back to my chair, picked up my backpack, and headed back to the condo. I wanted to erupt and confront Marie with what I just overheard from her friends. But I needed to keep quiet.

Every incident before the interaction at the pool could have had an explanation. The social worker could have been a support for Marie, a confidential appointment. Marie may have taken my father for more chemo after we stopped treatment because she loved him and wanted him to live longer. But again, it wasn't Marie's choice to make. I didn't understand why Marie accused me of being the no-good, money-chasing daughter to her friends. But by divine synchronicity, her friends had given me a clue.

One evening at the condo, Marie made dinner. Just enough for her and my father. She ate and talked with my father while I sat on the couch, and they watched TV. My father asked if I wanted some. I said no, thank you. Marie excluded me. She was sending me a message. Through her consistent attempts to shut me out, she gave me more reasons to stay and find out why she wanted to get rid of me.

Marie took my father out most of the day. He was exhausted when he returned home. As a result, I had little time with him. I needed help. This was getting to me, and I had another two weeks to go. So, I called home to the two people I knew who always had my back. I asked my brother and my husband if they could come down. Without hesitation, they both flew in the next day. Although they had separate flights, they arrived at the airport around the same time.

It was late afternoon, and I was sitting on the couch with Marie. She sat at an angle with her back to me, facing my father in his chair across the room. We were watching the early evening news. When my brother and Mark knocked, I answered the door. The second Marie saw them, she shot upright. As soon as my father saw them, he jumped up, walked towards them, and opened his arms wide to hug them. Marie avoided contact and sat in a chair across the living room, next to their bedroom door.

Marie didn't threaten to leave my father and shout ultimatums at him, like when I arrived. And she didn't greet them with her usual smile that showed all her teeth. Instead, her eyes grew wide, and she retreated.

Marie asked, "Why are you here?"

My brother said, "To visit Dad. He said we could come anytime to visit him. He told us we are always welcome."

We were all together. My father was so happy. My brother, Mark, and I stayed in the guest room. My brother slept on the floor. The next morning, Marie carried on with her usual routine. She took my father out early. When she left, I asked Mark to keep an eye out for when they returned. Then I asked my brother to help me explore everything of my father's as if it were a potential clue.

My next task was to follow up with his IRA. When I called, I was told that the notary had signed the document for the POA in the wrong place. I had already waited seven days. Now it was delayed for another seven to ten business days from the time they received it again, because of an error the notary at the bank made. My hard copy had to be mailed, no exceptions, which dragged the process out more. I needed to go back to the library. There I printed another form to bring to the bank. When I arrived at the bank, I made sure the notary signed it in the correct space. Lesson learned, from then on, I did not assume things were correct and in order. I checked, and triple-checked, every request I made.

In the meantime, I checked with local banks within a small radius of their home to see if any safe deposit boxes were in my father's name or jointly with another person. I had the hard copy of my power of attorney with me and the invoked letter of incapacitation and explained that I was doing my due diligence because there was a suspicion of theft and fraud.

Since I arrived in Florida, Marie acted suspiciously. She threatened my father and told her friends I was after my father's money. She was busy building alliances to push a judge's decision in her favor. Her friends' testimony was the ammunition she needed to gain control over my father. For nineteen years, Marie created the optics. She appeared to love my father and our family, but the truth was coming out and dismantling the illusion she configured. She revealed her feelings, and they were irrefutable.

LESSONS LEARNED

I believe financial opportunists, whether family members, caretakers, friends, spouses, or adult children, create their smoke screens by developing a pattern of theft within the account(s). Investigators look for withdrawals in large sums and deviations within a pattern in the account. However, theft is not always apparent when the exploiter has been in control and setting up the pattern of withdrawals of the account they are stealing from.

If there is a suspicion of fraud, theft, or extortion, my advice:

1. Block the threat.

2. Investigate after every financial account has been secured. Keep emotions in check and move quickly. By the time suspicion arises, more than likely, theft is occurring.

3. Contact financial institutions and request an investigation into the account. While they conduct their investigation, it will benefit you to conduct yours.

4. Contact the police and fill out a police report. If you believe that the financial threat is active, and you suspect it is a person whom you know, under no circumstances should you confront the person or alert them to your suspicion. Leave that to the police.

5. If the person with power of attorney has not been actively monitoring accounts, request a full history of financial statements.

6. To stop further theft of existing checking and savings accounts, close them out immediately and open new accounts with the power of attorney's name and title power of attorney on the account.

More financial safeguards and steps to investigate a financial account in the back of the book.

Chapter 14
Proof Wasn't Enough

It was the third week of March 2018 at the condo in Florida. Over a week went by and I was still waiting for the VA social worker to get back to me about my father's healthcare proxy he signed, naming Marie. My brother and Mark were with me when I called to follow up from the condo after Marie and my father left. The social worker hesitated when I said I asked to speak to my father's oncologist. I guessed what her answer would be after I waited for an extended hold.

The social worker said, "No, I cannot give you any information and I'm sorry, but the doctor is busy, and he cannot speak to you right now."

I left a message for him, hoping for a return call. As soon as I hung up, my brother, husband, and I went to the VA to retrieve my father's medical records. I needed an insight into what was going on. We arrived to find a maze of long lines and packed waiting areas. I took a numbered ticket, and we waited like everyone else. When we were called to the desk, I presented a copy of my invoked power of attorney, healthcare proxy, and ID. They took copies and I explained who I was, and my reason for being there. After waiting a few minutes, I was told there was no record of my father having a daughter, only a son. My brother requested my father's full medical record. I asked the woman behind the desk who I could talk to about my father's healthcare proxy, while we waited for the 362 pages to print. We were referred to the Office of Social Services.

On our way to their office, we passed waiting areas three and four deep with veterans. There were men in wheelchairs, some were

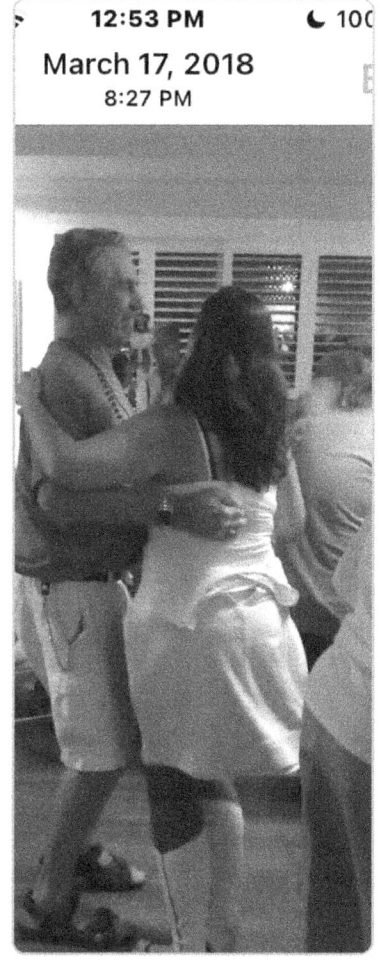

Jacqueline and her father at a Saint Patrick's Day party at the clubhouse in Florida, March 2018.
Photo by John Sullivan, used with permission

missing limbs, and others stood on crutches. The overflow of those who were waiting spilled over into the hallways where they lined the walls and wrapped around corners. Their eyes were fixed on the now-serving electronic board as they waited for their number to appear.

My brother and I waited in the Office of Social Services, only to be told, *I'm sorry I can't help you*. They sent us to the director. On our way there, we passed the same line and saw the same faces. They hadn't moved an inch.

I started reading my father's records, while we waited for the director. There were multiple visits to the emergency room since they came back to Florida, in November. Not a call, or text from Marie. Not one word when I called to ask her how my father was. She said she would return if my father's health got worse. By the number of emergency room visits and follow-ups, his health was worse. The progress reports noted that the wife made multiple phone calls to the hospital. As the reason for the visits, my father complained that…it's hard to breathe. He had trouble breathing and couldn't catch his breath. On one visit, they diagnosed him with severe bronchitis, COPD on another visit, and pneumonia on another. The scheduled appointments, ER visits, and the list of ailments went on and on. Marie was always in the background when I called my father from home. She made no mention of this, not even their ER visit on the day I arrived in Florida.

The office of medical records told me there was no mention of my father having a daughter. I don't know if my father's oncologist said this to prevent me from obtaining my father's records or if it was a clerical error. But the oncologist knew I existed because he documented it on page 271 of his 362-page medical record.

Each person I met at the VA had their version of an explanation of why my father received chemotherapy. I showed the director my father's original healthcare proxy and compared it to theirs. His medical visit notes from the VA contained one common denominator; my father understood what the treatment was and the course of treatment every single visit. It's hard to believe. Because, within a millisecond of explaining anything to my father, he'd ask three, four, and five times what he was doing. And he always wanted to know why.

The VA oncologist, nurse, and social workers never identified cognitive impairment. This was baffling to me. I showed the social services director the evaluation by his Alzheimer's physician dated before the healthcare proxy he signed at the VA. The Alzheimer's evaluation stated my father had considerable atrophy and his testing represented a significant interval decline. Meaning there was a substantial increase in his rate of decline.

The major discrepancies didn't faze the head of the social services department. And moments of clarity, as she described, were possible. Possible, yes. But one hundred percent of the time, every visit? It made little sense, yet they wanted me to believe that my father's gradual, consistent decline with increasing periods of memory lapses only occurred outside their hospital visits.

I pointed out the differences in their cognitive evaluation compared to my father's Alzheimer's evaluation back in Massachusetts before he left for Florida. My father's results from one evaluation were abnormal. In this category naming test, they showed pictures of animals, and he had to name as many as he could within a minute. In sixty seconds, he named nine. He also could not recall the three words said to him when he was asked after a brief time lapsed. In addition, when the Alzheimer's physician asked him what town he was in, he did not know. Nor did he remember what floor of the medical building he was on.

My father could not draw a clock with the numbers or position the hands to show a specific time. The VA oncologist's evaluation did not include these tests. His Alzheimer's physician noted he had two instances of *perseveration*, which means he repeated a particular response, and he could not transition or switch to a response that was appropriate according to the context of the question or subject.

The Alzheimer's physician conducted his evaluation of my father with him alone, whereas the VA oncologist allowed Marie to stay in the room while he conducted his cognitive assessment. I saw first-hand how my father answered questions by himself, contrary to when he was with Marie. She prompted him and he relied on her for cues on how to respond appropriately.

The director wanted us to bring my father in to test him. My brother and I told her there was no way we were putting my father through that. He was dying. He had stage 3b lung cancer and Alzheimer's. My father was beyond fatigued. He was dying and living the last 6 months of his life. His body and mind craved sleep. Yet he was run ragged for months, being schlepped back and forth to the VA hospital instead of being in home care. It wasn't right. Just the logistics of picking my father up, driving him to the VA, and him not understanding where he was going would have caused him agitation, frustration, and more confusion.

The director proposed a phone evaluation. My brother called our father, and he answered. He was home alone. It was a Wednesday and Marie was in her art class at the clubhouse. The director introduced herself to my father.

She asked him, "What day of the week is it? What year is it? Who is the president?"

My father said the wrong day. He stalled at the year and guessed at the president, which he got wrong. But that didn't change the director's opinion. She determined that the new healthcare proxy he signed at their VA would remain valid.

My father did not understand the healthcare proxy he signed at the VA with Marie by his side. He didn't remember he had Alzheimer's.

The VA physician, the oncologist nurse, and the social worker took their direction from Marie, not my father. Marie spoke for my father, and he followed her lead. He trusted her, and with her gentle suggestion, my father signed a new healthcare proxy. He had no memory or comprehension of what he signed.

The medical staff who cared for my father analyzed his capacity to understand based on how he looked, acted, and interacted with Marie and them. My father could not communicate the reason for his doctor's visit and the symptoms he was having. His medical intake was done with Marie by my father's side. She was the source of all my father's medical information, not him. Marie voiced her opinions and beliefs about what she wanted for my father's medical care and treatment to his physicians. And they abided by her decisions.

In the event of a court case, the VA attorneys would argue that chemotherapy and radiation caused no harm. It didn't matter that my father refused treatment that would extend his life if he had a terminal disease with no chance of a cure, in his original healthcare proxy. Furthermore, we agreed to end chemo and radiation as a family in Massachusetts and we reinstated my father's wishes. Marie was with us and included in the conversation.

My father should have been receiving mainly in-home care, and palliative care, at home months ago. It's called the continuum of care. This would have created a road map for medical personnel to follow and to see his changing needs along the progression of his Alzheimer's and lung cancer diseases. Palliative care ideally would have dovetailed into hospice care, making a more seamless transition.

I explained the entire story to each office I went into at the VA. They became stone-faced when I showed the major discrepancies between their evaluation and his Alzheimer's evaluation. I showed undeniable proof that their cognitive evaluation made the validity of their healthcare proxy naming Marie questionable. They listened, but nothing I said made any difference.

LESSON LEARNED

The fact is, my father's Alzheimer's evaluation was not the same as his oncologist's. In scientific methods of research studies, it boils down to this: two different cognitive test evaluations, two methods of testing, and two different standard procedures resulted in two different cognitive assessments. The Alzheimer's physician was not qualified to evaluate my father's cancer, and the oncologist was not a neurologist trained in degenerative diseases of the brain.

Shouldn't a physician specialized in the field of Alzheimer's make the final decision on evaluations? Especially when determining if a person with Alzheimer's can understand, fill out, and sign legal documents. I think so, but it's not how the system works.

DURABLE POWER OF ATTORNEY
OF
JOHN J. SULLIVAN

KNOW ALL MEN BY THESE PRESENTS:

That I, **JOHN J. SULLIVAN**, presently of _____ Florida, constitute and appoint **JACQUELINE J. SULLIVAN-WYCO**, presently of Hubbardston, Massachusetts, my true and lawful attorney for me and in my name, place and stead and on my behalf to act under the following provisions:

1. General Powers. To exercise or perform any act, power, duty, right or obligation whatsoever that I now have or may hereafter acquire, relating to any person, matter, transaction or property, real or personal, tangible or intangible, now owned or hereafter acquired by powers granted below. I further grant to my said attorney full power and authority to do everything necessary in exercising any of the powers herein granted as fully as I might or could do if personally present, except as provided in § 709.08, Florida Statutes, or any successor provision of law, excluding § 709.08(7)(b)(5).

John J. Sullivan
JOHN J. SULLIVAN

2. Powers of Collection and Payment. To demand, sue for, collect, compromise, recover and receive all debts, moneys, property interests, claims and demands whatsoever, now due or that may hereafter be or become due to me, including the right to institute any legal or equitable proceedings therefore; and to execute and deliver on my behalf and in my name, any and all endorsements, releases, receipts, and discharges for the same.

John J. Sullivan
JOHN J. SULLIVAN

3. Banking Powers. To make, execute, deliver and endorse notes, drafts, checks, certificates of deposit and orders for the payment of money or other property from or to me in order of my name; to open or close bank accounts or any other investment accounts; the right to make deposits or withdrawals on any and all accounts in banks or other financial institutions on my behalf, and generally exercise control over such accounts. I grant my attorney authority to conduct banking transactions as provided in § 709.2208(1), Florida Statutes, as well as authority to conduct investment transactions as provided in § 709.2208(2), Florida Statutes. I authorize my attorney to execute any form, power of attorney, required by any bank or other financial institution in order to enable my attorney in fact to execute the powers granted under this instrument.

Records from the author. *Image of this document is the property of Jacqueline Sullivan Wyco, who had power of attorney for her father.*

Chapter 15
In the Eyes of Judgment

In general, as human beings, we form hundreds of subjective opinions of people whom we interact with daily. These opinions and feelings about others are based on our history, beliefs, and experiences.

Consciously and unconsciously, we read and calculate hundreds of microfacial, and physical expressions, and situational interactions we have with a person. Their hygiene, how they dress, talk, don't talk, interact, gender, non-gender, mannerisms, their relationships, the color of their skin, ethnic background, clothing, personality, job, or no job, home, or no home status, addictions, and habits. You name it, we judge it.

We make an assessment about a person, in a fraction of a second, with no background on a person, and no framework, other than what we see. Furthermore, on the other end of the spectrum, one's opinion of a person can also be influenced by another person's opinion or experience with that person. And this applies to professionals, such as medical staff and attorneys, as well as everyday people. In conclusion, we cannot say with complete confidence that our judgments of others are correct without having all the facts to make an objective assessment.

In March 2018, there was a party coming up for Saint Patrick's Day at the clubhouse in the condo community in Florida. Marie had bought tickets for her and my father. She said if my brother, my husband, and I wanted to go, we should call Murray, my father's friend. It appeared the rift had blown over.

When we walked down to Murray's to pick up the tickets, there was no sign of a past feud. He never mentioned it. I had known Murray for over thirty years, from when my father was transferred to Ladder 7 in Meetinghouse Hill. Murray and his wife lived on the Cape in the summer across from my house, in a seasonal campground. He was a friend of my father and our family. If there was a rift, he would have mentioned it. He was the type of person who cleared the air, so there were no misunderstandings. My father was the same. They both worked to solve problems. It's what Murray did professionally as a stress counselor, after the fire department.

While my brother, Mark, and I were there, we brought up Marie. We went over everything that had recently transpired. He said he didn't know what to say, because she was his friend, too. Then, I told Murray about the time when my father called me looking for Marie.

I said, "Dad called me. He had just woken up and was looking for Marie. When I called her phone, she said she was at Target, shopping."

I knew Marie had routinely left my father to wait on a bench in front of the store while she shopped. She half chuckled when she told me about the time he wandered to the other side of the store where she found him talking to someone. It scared me enough that I ordered a Brickhouse Security GPS tracker. The chain of emails with Marie dates to November 2017. I told her I could help her set it up. She declined. I found it in a kitchen drawer in the condo, still in its original packaging. The cord was snugged tight in the box. It was never unraveled.

Murray didn't seem surprised. He told me Marie had gone out several times in the mornings and left my father home alone because it was easier for her. Leaving my father at home alone was her way of doing errands. My father wandered before, but that didn't concern Marie. She could have had a neighbor stay with my father while she ran out or used the GPS device to alert her if my father wandered past a pre-set boundary. But she didn't.

By this time, my brother and I weren't sure what to do or who to call anymore. We didn't know if we should file a police report. Leaving my father on a bench and home alone was dangerous but it wasn't considered a crime. Marie threatened to leave him, but she would deny it and my father had already forgotten. We didn't see how filling out a report was going to help us.

An investigation might take weeks. A surprise visit from elder services was not going to reveal anything in a brief encounter. They didn't know there was more behind Marie's smile and welcoming demeanor. She portrayed the doting wife and caretaker, but it didn't always reflect the person she was when she was alone with my father. By nature, my father was well-mannered and cooperative, and their home was clean, organized, and maintained. There's nothing in the appearance of my father, Marie, or their home for an investigator to believe that he had suffered or was suffering in any way.

We called our attorney back home with whom we had on retainer and set up a date for a conference call. We feared for my father's safety. I sounded unhinged. I know I did. I emailed our attorney about my concern before our call. We asked if we could move my father from Florida back to Massachusetts, ship his vehicle home, and move his belongings out of their Cape home.

We were told yes, but instructed to think carefully, as we should consider our relationship with Marie's daughter, her trustee, who owned the other half of the Cape home. Our attorney advised if I moved my father and his belongings, I could strain the relationship, that I needed to be on good terms for future communications, and that I should think twice before taking any action. Our attorney downplayed my concerns about my father's safety and well-being. To her, I was like the crazed daughter who had it out for her stepmother, the classic rivalry.

When the call ended, we sat there, deflated. Everything had turned upside down and we couldn't figure it out. The more we tried to advocate for my father, the more discouraged we became.

After the conference call, the three of us needed a time-out. We took a drive by the water, to have a drink. We didn't talk much. We mostly just stared out at the Atlantic Ocean. My father signed IRA checks. He didn't sell the stocks, withdraw the money, or change direct deposit to paper checks. He didn't drive himself to the bank. But what did that prove? My father had Alzheimer's and leaving him at home alone could be considered negligent, but who would come forward and testify? And aside from that, it wasn't a crime for a wife to make her husband's medical care decisions, even if it wasn't what he wanted or legally set up. Marie's marriage to my father gave her total control. There were no signs of physical abuse, and I couldn't prove coercion or mental torment, even though I witnessed it.

⌘⌘⌘

Marie sat across from me at the Saint Patrick's Day party with my husband and brother at the same table. Everyone at the party was laughing, smiling, and moving about, but not Marie. She looked irritated. She glared at me as she talked with her friends who sat beside her. She kept her voice down. I couldn't hear what she was saying to them, but I caught the look they gave me as they were listening to her. I sat next to my father's best friend, Murray.

Murray said, "It's good to see your father out."

I said, "What do you mean?"

Murray said, "Marie stopped coming to functions at the clubhouse with your father. He hasn't been down here in a long time. It's too bad because he loves being around people."

I wasn't aware of this. Marie had made it sound like they were still active socially in the community. And in the past, they had signed up for almost every event. My father lit up when he was around friends. His body synced with the rhythm as soon as the music started at any party. He couldn't listen to music without moving with the beat. He was light on his feet and when we danced that night, his Alzheimer's seemed to disappear.

Murray's comment enlightened me to what life was really like for my father. People are born social beings, and this makes isolation so debilitating. The consistent withdrawal of socialization alters the mind, the body, and the spirit.

My father's social interaction mainly came from going to the VA hospital, the emergency room, and other visits to doctors. Yes, people surrounded him, but not in an environment that fostered pure happiness and joy, and not by people who knew and loved him. There's a difference. We all need and crave meaningful connections with each other, but Marie, by design, kept my father away from his friends and family. The distance Marie created between my father, our family, and his friends, caused social deprivation.

LESSON LEARNED
When is controlling a person's interactions determined as abuse? The answer lies in the pattern. "Pulling away a person from their network makes them reliant on their partner. In coercive control, the abuser monitors and controls the victim's communication and interactions with others. In turn, the victim becomes increasingly isolated from friends, family, and other social connections."31 From Verywell Mind, 4 Early Signs of Coercive Control.

⸺⸺⸺

The day after the party, I continued to work on securing my father's finances. My brother and I finally got my father's IRA moved, but that came with unforeseen delays and hurdles. Initially, the day we drove to a bank branch to file my power of attorney paperwork. I explained to the customer service representative that my father had Alzheimer's, and I wanted to move his account laterally because there was a suspicion of theft. She informed me it would take a couple of days to process and that she'd get back to us. We waited only to be told that there may be a problem because Florida state laws had changed and updated, and it affected my ability to move my father's IRA even though I was his power of attorney. (Therefore, I recommend advocates review state laws once a year.) She said she would call to get more information, and she'd get back to us as soon as she had an answer. She was one of the few people who went to bat for us.

One evening shortly thereafter, while we were sitting and talking with my father, Marie asked us, "Why did you move your father's IRA? I would never touch it."

I offered no information to Marie about my father's IRA. Yet, she felt compelled to reveal she knew it was moved. Furthermore, she proclaimed that she would never touch it. Marie had no reason to access my father's IRA. She had full access to his checking account, to which his pension and Social Security were directly deposited.

It is important to note here that no financial institution may reveal private information unless the account owner has granted permission. The financial institution didn't screen my father for Alzheimer's. In addition, there is no training that I know of for phone representatives on Alzheimer's and how to detect coercion. Handling a person's life savings comes with few effective security screening measures over the phone.

I witnessed for years how Marie, with the slightest nudge, prompted my father to answer questions during his Alzheimer's. In theory, all my father had to do was reply *YES* to the customer service representative when they asked him if he would allow Marie to be a user on his account. Marie wasn't the beneficiary or the power of attorney. Nor was his IRA jointly owned by her. I didn't have time to investigate the losses, but I suspected checks were being mailed to the condo.

In 2016, my father didn't recall what day it was or know what zip code he was in. My father didn't own a computer or have an email address. If he did make a call to his financial institution with automated prompts, he couldn't follow the instructions, let alone conduct an online transaction.

My brother and I weren't sure how to protect my father. We called the attorney who drew up my father's directives. They had offices in both Florida and Massachusetts. The office in Massachusetts told us to call the Florida office. The Florida office said they needed to look into it and call the attorney who drew up the original documents before I could ask questions. After a follow-up call with them, we were told there was a conflict of interest and that they could not provide me with any further information because my father and Marie both used the same attorney to draw up their irrevocable trusts, homesteads, healthcare proxy, living will, and last wills and testaments.

Shouldn't the attorney who drew up my father's directives be able to speak to me, considering I was his named advocate? Another door had closed on us, but I kept searching.

I found an attorney who we met in Palm Beach. He was gritty, to say the least, and he postured himself as an aggressive, no-nonsense litigator. He stood as he talked to me, my brother, and my husband, sitting at the conference table. The lion mural took up the entire wall behind him. It was a statement. As I was talking, he cut me off. He didn't need or want to hear the details of my story, and he could have cared less about the pile of documents I had. He was the type of attorney you'd want in your corner. Time is money, and he didn't waste it. He told me I needed to decide. If we wanted to take my father home to Massachusetts, he said we needed to go for guardianship. He said he didn't come cheap, $10,000 minimum to start. The process to obtain guardianship was based on a judge's decision from a trial with testimony from witnesses called on both sides.

Marie created a persona of who I was. She convinced her friends I was stealing from my father. As for the professionals, social workers, and the physicians Marie brought him to, she said that what I wanted for my father was not what he wanted. It wasn't true. But they didn't know me. There would be nothing more convincing to the court than testimony told by people who believed Marie's every word.

We had Murray, maybe, but he already told me Marie was his friend, too. Murray was stuck in the middle, and he didn't want to be there. The judge's decision could go either way.

On the way back to the condo from the attorney, we stopped for a coffee to discuss our options. Guardianship wasn't the answer. The odds were against me, and people's misperception of me would overshadow the truth. I knew it and I feared we'd lose. If we did, we might never see my father again.

One option was to take him. That is what the woman at the bank suggested when we told her our story. She had a similar situation with a friend's son years prior.

She said, "Just get him in the car and drive."

A solution, but at what cost? I didn't want to give Marie a reason to call the police. She wanted to get rid of me and she flipped facts and turned the truth faster than I could say my full name. I heard how convincing she was. Her friends at the pool believed her rendition of me as a daughter. To the police, it probably didn't matter that I was my father's invoked proxy, and I could legally move him. Marie was fighting it and had friends to vouch for her. And we didn't need an all-points bulletin alert out on us. My brother and my husband had to leave in a few days, and I was missing them already. We decided the best thing to do was for me to stay until the end of the month, as I had originally planned.

After my father's death, I investigated his account and discovered letters of confirmation changes made to his Vanguard account dated February 8, 2016. Another letter confirmed Marie's email and phone number, which had been added to his account. In another letter, Marie wrote *CONFIRMED* at the top of the beneficiary page. She dated it 4/27/16. Then I found the Vanguard confirmation of account changes with a check payable to the new address on record. My father's Florida address.

My father's out-of-the-blue statement to Marie, "Didn't we just get a check" wasn't a figment of his imagination. His moment of clarity was a window of truth. He had been receiving, signing, and cashing many Vanguard checks. The note in the trash from the postwoman addressed to Marie, "I will continue to hold Jack's mail," confirmed that Marie didn't want me to see the IRA check that was expected to arrive at his home while I was there that month. There was no record of where the cash went.

LESSON LEARNED

Committing fraud and theft is as easy as making a phone call by the exploiter and yes said over the phone by a person with Alzheimer's. I suggest that the person who has power of attorney:

- Be present when the person signs their advanced directives. If not physically, by Facetime or Zoom.
- Remove all financial information from your loved one's place of residence.
- Change usernames, passwords, email, and mailing address on all financial accounts.
- Monitor all accounts at a minimum of once a month.
- Send the power of attorney and letter of incapacitation documents

overnight for investment companies.

- Confirm beneficiaries and POA contact information with the company by phone and email.
- Show the notary where to sign documents. Sending documents with a signature in the incorrect place causes delays in securing and investigating the account.
- Make all required minimum distributions (RMD) direct deposit.
- Although paper checks are traceable, once one is signed and cashed, it's gone. Furthermore, it is not always possible to get a copy of the back of a check that's been signed. I was told by Vanguard I needed a subpoena, but even then it wasn't guaranteed. However, there is a way.

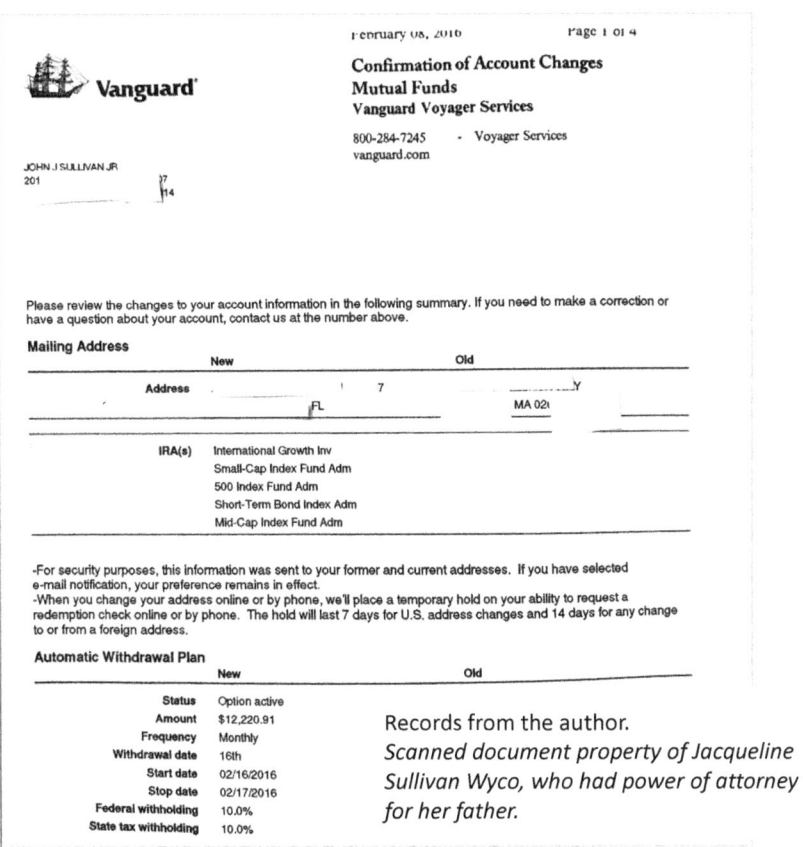

Records from the author.
Scanned document property of Jacqueline Sullivan Wyco, who had power of attorney for her father.

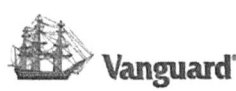

Confirmation of Account Changes
Mutual Funds
Vanguard Voyager Services

February 08, 2010   Page 2 of 4

JOHN J SULLIVAN JR

800-284-7245 - Voyager Services
vanguard.com

Automatic Withdrawal Plan (Continued)

	New	Old
Check payable to	Address of record	-

IRA(s)		
	International Growth Inv	
	$2,444.18	
	Small-Cap Index Fund Adm	
	$2,444.18	
	500 Index Fund Adm	
	$2,444.19	
	Short-Term Bond Index Adm	
	$2,444.18	
	Mid-Cap Index Fund Adm	
	$2,444.18	
Total	$12,220.91	

- If the date you specified falls on a weekend or holiday, we will process the transaction on the preceding business day.
If you've taken an early or premature distribution from your retirement plan, Vanguard will update your tax status

Records from the author
Scans of the document above and those on the facing page, are the property of Jacqueline Sullivan Wyco, who had power of attorney for her father.

In the Eyes of Judgment

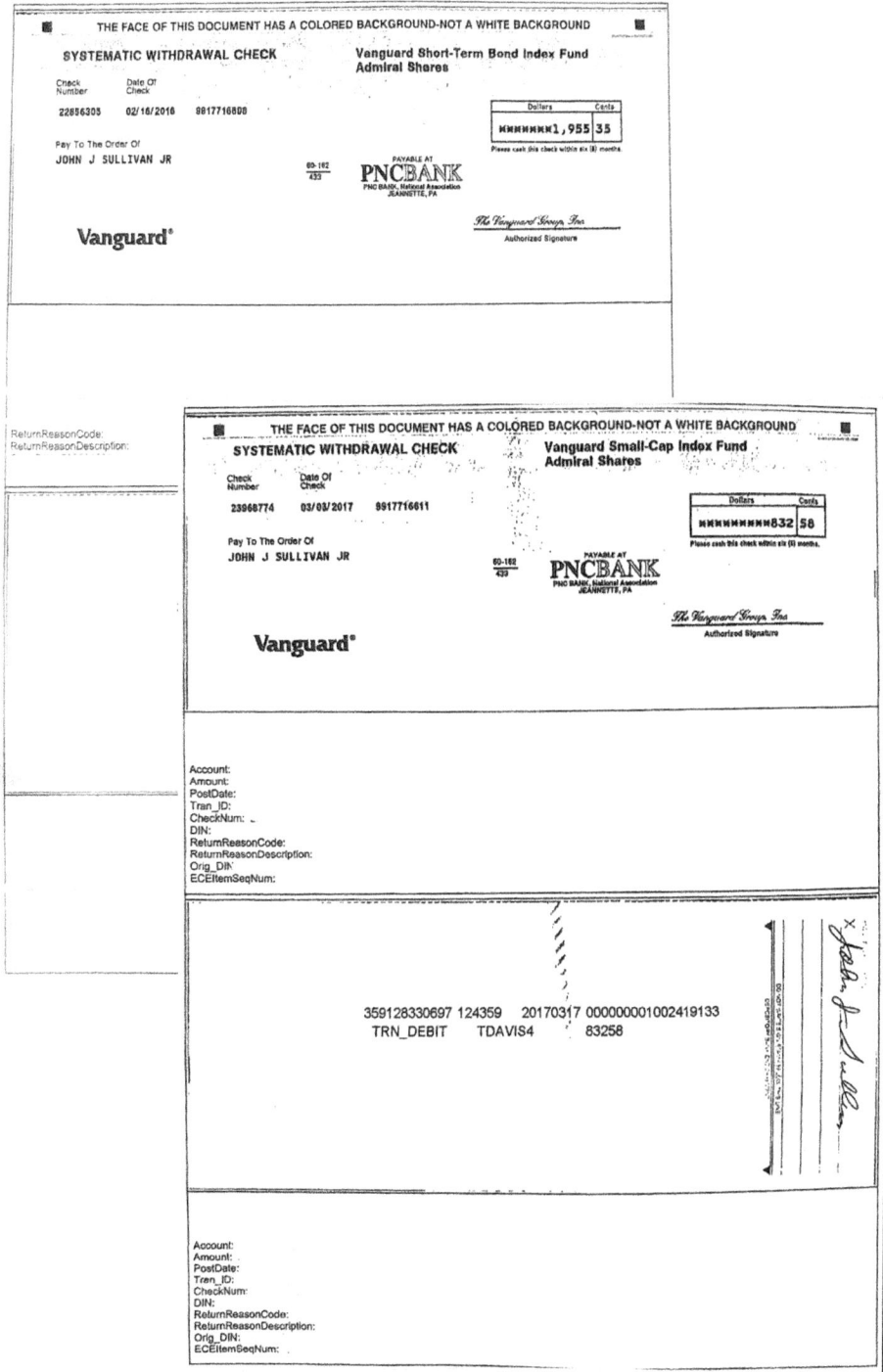

139

Fear Knocked   — Jacqueline Sullivan Wyco

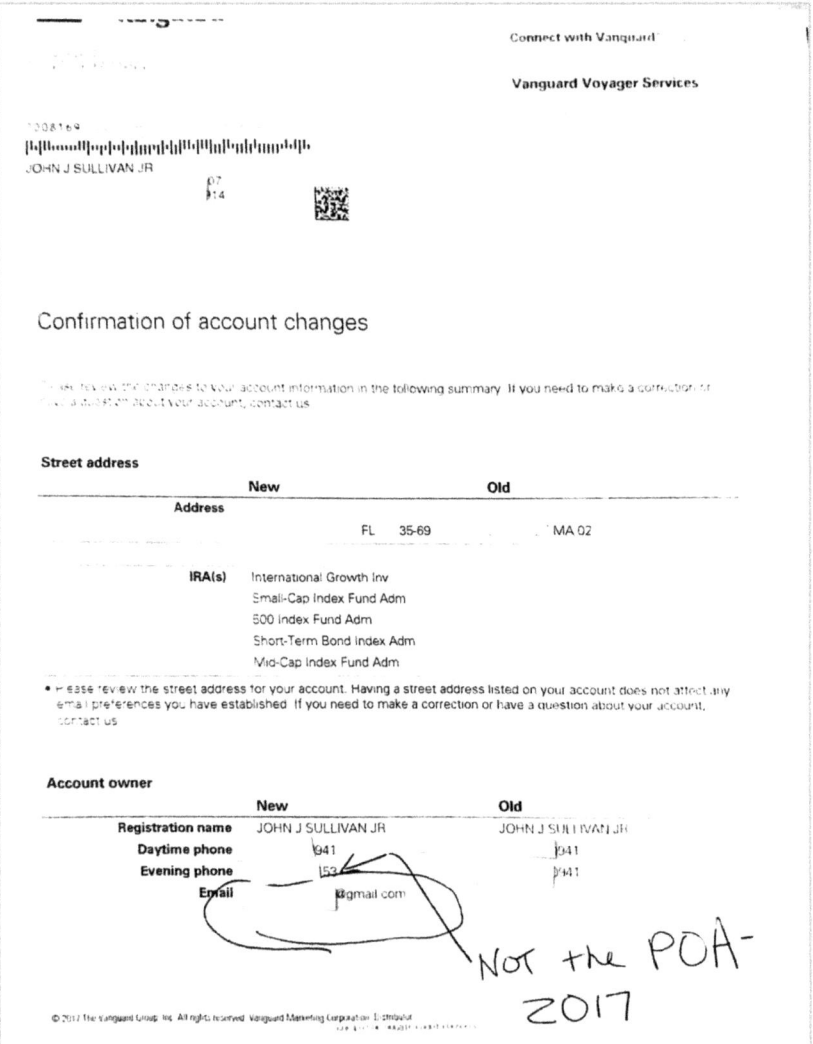

Records from the author
Scans of the document above and those on the facing page, are the property of Jacqueline Sullivan Wyco, who had power of attorney for her father.

March 0?, 2016

Beneficiary Verification
Vanguard Voyager Services

Vanguard

800-284-7245 • Voyager Services
vanguard.com

4/27/16
Confirmed

...ur beneficiary designations

...you. We're sending this reminder to ensure that the beneficiary designations for your Vanguard ... to date.

...at we have accurate information, because your beneficiary designations generally determine who ...ccounts and may supersede the information in your will or trust. You should review and update your ...gnations whenever you experience a major life event, such as a birth, marriage, divorce, or death.

...n below is correct, you don't need to take any action. Just file this document with your records.

...hange your designations, you can do so in one of the following ways:

...to your account at vanguard.com; from the "My Accounts" dropdown, select "Account maintenance"; then ...profile," choose "Beneficiaries."

RAs, call us at the number above to update your beneficiaries. For nonretirement accounts, ...s, and 403(b)(7)s, call us at the number above to request the appropriate form.

...not able to accept any beneficiary changes marked on this document.

eneficiaries

	Name	Birth/Trust Date	Allocation
Primary	JACQUELINE SULLIVAN WYCO		50.00%
	JOHN SULLIVAN		50.00%
Primary Total			100.00%
Secondary	You haven't designated any beneficiaries of this type. Please read important information below regarding the distribution of your assets upon your death.		
econdary Total			100.00%

Chapter 16
Patterns Emerge

My brother and Mark went home, and during my month-long stay in March 2018, Marie prepared to leave Florida. She shredded documents, packed, and shipped many of her belongings home to the Cape. In the four rooms of the condo, the only thing left on the walls were the faded outlines of the framed oil canvases she had painted from photos she took in Greece, Spain, and other European destinations.

The three of us were scheduled to fly out of Florida, a couple of days after Marie's art show. There was a noticeable decline in my father over the past four weeks. He had grown more confused, had little energy, and fell asleep routinely in his chair after sitting only a few minutes. I didn't know how my father would do on the plane. The process of getting to the airport and on the plane could trigger agitation. How much? I didn't know. In the twenty minutes leading up to our ride to the airport, my stomach tied itself in knots and my head pounded. My father asked where we were going several times.

Marie opened the front door while she finished packing her last bag. I carried the rest of the luggage downstairs. My father's friend who lived in the same building upstairs from him, yelled up to Marie from the parking lot below. He said he loved her and my dad. She returned the sentiment. He was a nice guy from New York, a retired cop. My father liked him and his wife, and he referred to him as a great guy. He seemed to care very much for my father and Marie, but he looked at me sideways. By his look, I knew Marie had shared the same narrative with him as she did the two ladies down at the pool.

I arranged for my father's car to be transported on the same day we were coming home. He and Marie wouldn't return to the condo. And I didn't know when I could get back to Florida. My father no longer drove, and he began leaving his car in Florida because they flew home when I didn't drive them. Marie had her vehicle down on the Cape. On our way to the airport and inside the terminal, my father kept asking where we were going. He grew anxious, and fidgety as we sat in the plane on the tarmac.

The man in front of him reclined his seat as far as it would go, and the back of his seat hit my father's knees. My father squeezed into his seat with his legs sideways facing the aisle. During the flight, my father looked as if he were on the edge of a meltdown. If I had waited even another week, I may not have been able to get him on a flight at all. Marie planned for their ride home to the Cape and when we landed, I walked them over to their pickup location and asked her to text me to let me know they got home alright, which she did.

Marie called me the following morning. Her phone was on the speaker. My father listened in the background.

She said, "The car is missing. I think I should call the police."

I said, "The car has been shipped home. Like I explained before I went down."

She asked, "Where's the title?"

I said, "I have it."

Marie sounded bewildered and I sensed her gritting her teeth.

She said, "I don't appreciate that you took the car without consulting me."

I said, "But I did."

Marie repeated to my father, "Jacqueline took the car and it's on its way back from Florida."

He said, "Okay."

I repeated, "Dad, your car is on a transport carrier on the way back from Florida."

Marie asked specifically for the title. She didn't need the title to drive his car if it was what she wanted to do. The title of ownership is required for only two things, either to buy or sell a vehicle.

I talked with my brother when I got off the phone with her and my father. In hindsight, we were relieved we didn't take my father home without her knowing, because now we knew she would have called the police in a heartbeat.

My husband and I visited my father on the Cape about a week later. While we were there, Marie reminded my father his car was gone. He did not want to give up driving and the freedom he associated with it. Revoking his driver's license had caused him such immense agitation before, but Marie wound him up nevertheless and it sent him reeling.

I waited until my father went to the bathroom.

I said, "Marie, I'm not doing this. I am not here to fight."

Marie created a drama surrounding the car. It should have been a non-issue, but Marie's pattern of behavior emerged. Marie lashed out through my father when I didn't give her what she wanted on demand. My father didn't understand it was her way of getting back. I thought her angered burst was done and over with when I left that day, but I was mistaken.

When I went home, later that evening, I got six phone calls. The first couple I answered. My father yelled into the phone.

He said, "Jacqueline, it's Dad. I want the papers for my car! I want them now!"

Then he hung up. This wasn't him talking. My father couldn't remember, during this time, where he put his phone, or have enough memory to remember why he called from the time he pressed the contact button to the time I answered the call. Marie's pattern had grown more predictable. And so was my father's because of the disease. Although I can't say with certainty that Marie called and put the words in my father's mouth. I can tell you that Marie didn't call or text me or my brother to ask us for help to diffuse the situation.

It was so bad, that after the third call, I stopped answering and let it go to voicemail. My father grew more furious and enraged with every call. I got texts from my brother. My father called and screamed at him because he wanted the tools he borrowed, returned.

I witnessed Marie in Florida when she tried to make my father tell me to leave. She expressed her rage toward me by using my father to do it. She didn't hide the fact that she wanted to divide us. My brother and I didn't respond to my father. It would have made the situation worse. Marie never attempted to de-escalate the situation among us.

And even though I knew my father's anger wasn't coming from him, it ripped me apart.

The transport truck delivered my father's car to my house. I sold it, and put the funds into his account for his care, after I checked with our attorney. Mark followed me to the dealership, the day I turned it in. Before I handed the keys over, I took down the two American flags and the Boston Fire sticker he had in the rear window. I choked up when the man helping me removed his Marine Corps license plate and handed it to me. When I went to thank him, I couldn't speak. It was more than just a car. It was a symbol. My father's life was coming to an end. I still had the lump in my throat when I left the dealership to get into the car with Mark. As he drove away, I turned the rear mirror and watched my father's car until I couldn't see it anymore. I felt like I was burying him, piece by piece.

My father had been getting worse by the day while Marie focused on getting the title to my father's car to prove ownership. Ironically, Marie had been talking about her next vehicle before this in Florida.

She said, "My next car is going to be loaded. It's going to have all the bells and whistles."

Our hearts were breaking. My father was dying from lung cancer. And Marie was excited and looking forward to purchasing a new car. Her focus didn't match up with what was happening in our lives, but again, that was Marie.

LESSONS LEARNED

I did what my father permitted me to do as his advocate. And I had to ask myself, why did this enrage Marie? And why anger my father and use it against me to persuade me to give her the title to his car? It didn't make sense. I should have taken this as a warning sign of a more serious pattern of behavior. "The goal of coercive control is to dominate the victim's thoughts, emotions, and actions through manipulation, intimidation, and various forms of emotional and psychological abuse to gain power and control over their partner."[32] From Verywell Mind, 4 Early Signs of Coercive Control.

Chapter 17
By Willful Omission

I urge every healthcare advocate to accompany the person with Alzheimer's to all their medical appointments, in person or via Facetime or Zoom because a healthcare proxy cannot ensure that a person's decisions will be honored by their physician.

After reading my father's medical notes, I saw Marie's narrative playing out just as it had back in Florida. There were several appointments and chronic health emergencies my father experienced at the VA in West Palm Beach, Florida, which me and my brother were unaware of. My father entrusted me with his care, yet Marie kept me out of the loop. During our conversations, she omitted every medical detail I discovered in his medical records. My father's rapid decline left my brother and me wondering if he should be living with her.

I investigated long-term care near both of our houses. I toured them and met with the directors and owners of the facilities. One place I visited was the same memory care facility where my father-in-law lived. He had dementia. I was told I could put a deposit on a room they had available, but the executive director asked that I bring my father in for an evaluation. I asked my brother what he thought. He said he could take him there. I told him the meeting would be informal, in the dining room where they would serve him lunch and ask him some preliminary questions to assess his needs.

It was a Friday when my brother picked our father up. He drove an hour out to the memory care facility where my husband and I met them. If we felt this was the right place for him, we planned on informing Marie afterward with the help of the director. I explained

> **Name:** John Sullivan   **Today's Date:** 08/21/17   **Last Visit Date:** 07/11/17
> **Referring PCP:** Julia ——— M.D.   **Office Location:** Plymouth
> **DOB:** 03/05/39   **Age:** 78 year   **Gender:** male   **SSN:** ———
>
> **Accompanied By:** Wife — ———   Daughter — Jacqueline, Son-in-law — Mark
>
> **Presenting Problem(s):**
> Alzheimer's disease with late onset: ICD10 = G30.1 / ICD9 = 331.0 / SNOMED = 416975007
>
> **Diagnoses (Problem List):**
> Alzheimer's disease with late onset ICD10 = G30.1 / ICD9 = 331.0 / SNOMED = 416975007
> Asthma ICD10 = J45.909 / ICD9 = 493.90 / SNOMED = 195967001
> Depression NOS ICD10 = F32.9 / ICD9 = 311 / SNOMED = 35489007
> Diverticulosis ICD10 = K57.90 / ICD9 = 562.10 / SNOMED = 397881000
> Hearing loss ICD10 = H91.90 / ICD9 = 389.9 / SNOMED = 15188001
> Hyperlipidemia ICD10 = E78.5 / ICD9 = 272.4 / SNOMED = 55822004
> Impingement syndrome of left shoulder ICD10 = M75.42 / ICD9 = 726.2 / SNOMED = 239960007
> Insomnia ICD10 = G47.00 / ICD9 = 780.52 / SNOMED = 193462001
>
> **Interventions at Last Visit:**
> At last visit, MMSE had declined to 18/30, category fluency to 10 animals in a minute, both representing a significant interval decline. At baseline, he had some excessive flatus, urinary frequency and rhinorrhea. He was to get his last dose of chemotherapy the next day with reassessment of response in the near future. He did have a local oncologist. I didn't see a definite changes cognitive capacity although was a remain positive and upbeat. I suspected the cognitive decline related to cessation of rivastigmine patch. He did have some rhinorrhea at baseline and urinary frequency even before being placed on cholinesterase inhibitors. I thought it was worthwhile to try him on a titration of galantamine ER (fair amount of local site reaction, concomitant with allergic reaction one of his chemotherapy agents).
>
> Point of cognition, think we do have some measure stabilization. I would like to add in memantine to see if we get a further boost and cognition. He is on the cusp between mild and moderate disease so I think it reasonable to try. He will be started on memantine. 10 mg size pills have been provided which may be broken in half for the titration for 5 mg dosings. Dosing will be 5 mg. each morning for Week 1, then 5 mg. twice per day for Week 2, then 10-5 mg. twice/day for Week 3, then 10 mg. twice/day starting and continuing at Week 4. Potential side effects were discussed as infrequent and usually mild. The most common of these are constipation, dizziness, confusion, headache. If any side effects are significant, I am to be contacted. I requested caregiver attention to any behavioral or cognitive changes after the Namenda has been started.
>
> Psychologically, I think he is doing fairly well with modest dose of sertraline. I'm certainly willing to prescribe it. I don't think he needs to see a psychopharmacologist independently at this point. We discussed some issues regarding health care proxy, power of attorney, living will. I think all concerned and the family have his interest at heart. There are some negotiations as to details that will occur.
>
> **Plan:**
>   Medication Changes:
>
> Printed On: 08/21/2017   Page 3 of 4

Medical Record obtained by Jacqueline, the designated healthcare proxy for her father, July 11, 2017

my dynamic with Marie and the most recent history of events with my father to the director. I also asked if she would arrange for a caretaker to accompany my father when Marie visited, and she agreed.

The director based her professional opinion on my father from the nurse's assessment, her observation, and her interaction with him.

She said, "From everything you've told me and by your father's assessment, I believe he belongs in memory care, not with Marie. I think you may need guardianship. I know a couple of local attorneys here in Worcester. I can give you their contact info if you'd like."

In my father's power of attorney, he named me in the event a judge had to decide who should take care of his medical and financial needs. It benefited him to have this clause in case another person petitioned the court for guardianship. But a family member is not always appointed. A judge can appoint a guardian from the court.

My brother and I met with the attorney the director referred us to. We brought all my father's advanced directives that outlined his long-term care decisions. We decided not to pursue guardianship because the attorney stated I already had legal authority.

My brother and I were still unsure about admitting my father into the long-term care facility. We felt an overwhelming sense of guilt. I know how much he feared nursing homes. We hadn't discussed this early on with him. I wasn't sure how he would react in a locked ward environment. My brother and I decided we would make it work so he could stay in his own home with Marie. But in doing so, we needed to hire a caretaker in his home.

I canceled the lease for his room and removed his belongings from the memory care facility in early April. Then I began working on hiring a person to go to his home regularly to monitor him on the Cape.

LESSON LEARNED

I didn't label Marie's actions against my father as abuse, harm, or neglect to the executive director. I didn't believe that the harm Marie caused was intentional, at first. I thought her behavior and actions were the result of the toll my father's disease was taking on her. It became clearer to me after the research I discovered. "There is a tendency to treat abuse as unintentional harm or neglect, thanks to a general assumption that families and partners always act with compassion towards the older person. Yet, the reality is often far from the idealized picture we have of care and support in later life."[33] From The Conversation, "The Combination of Dementia and Domestic Abuse Is All Too Often Overlooked."

On Saturday, April 21, 2018, I drove down to the Cape, to my father's and Marie's home, to meet with the hospice nurse for an evaluation. Even though his Alzheimer's physician recommended my father to be in hospice, he still needed to be evaluated. The hospice nurse asked if my father had a do-not-resuscitate order (DNR) and explained the Medical Orders for Life-Sustaining Treatment form. Patients like my father who are in hospice have these posted on their refrigerators instructing medical personnel who are called to the home, not to use any life-saving measures to save them. We had neither.

The hospice nurse took my father's vitals and asked Marie some general questions, such as how my father was sleeping and his appetite. She wanted to know, overall, how he was doing. Marie followed up by informing the nurse that the day before, on the 20th, an ambulance transported him to the hospital.

I asked Marie, "Why didn't you call me?"

She shrugged her shoulders and sighed.

She said, "You were going to be here today. You're finding out now."

I informed the hospice nurse of his invoked healthcare proxy, and that I was my father's advocate. At the end of the meeting, she told me that my father did not meet the strict criteria needed to qualify for hospice.

I pursued finding an in-home care company. Finally, after a couple of weeks, I received a referral for a visiting nurse company after several calls to patient advocacy for help. But there were still appointments my father had gone to with the primary care physician that neither she nor Marie communicated to me about. It was an ongoing battle to receive information. The Alzheimer's physician suggested a social worker for us, just as I did. I wanted peaceful visits with my father, and not to be involved in arguments with Marie.

On May 10, 2018, I emailed Marie to inform her I was working on getting a nurse and an aide into their home. I asked to discuss this over the phone, without having the speaker on with my father in the room.

On May 21, 2018, I went down to my father's house for the initial visit of the nurse. Marie sat at the kitchen table when I explained to the nurse I wanted updates after their visits, which she agreed to.

After the nurse went over each medication with Marie, she asked why the memantine prescription had a substantial number of pills left in the bottle. Marie had been told by the nurse he needed to take them twice daily, the required dosage prescribed on the bottle. Marie acknowledged she was aware of the dosage. She knew what the medication was for, yet she didn't give it to him.

The memantine was the Alzheimer's drug for memory enhancement. It was prescribed on August 21, 2017, by his Alzheimer's physician. I was at the appointment with Marie, and my husband Mark when he went over the dosage with her and us. Marie took it upon herself to cut it in half. Memantine wasn't a cure. It didn't stop or reverse Alzheimer's, it helped to improve memory and awareness. Because the nurse corrected Marie, I thought she'd give him the accurate dosage. But I found out two months later, that she had continued to cut his memory enhancement dosage in half.

My father's cognitive impairment was severely impaired during the last five months of his life. Marie drove and took my father everywhere including his primary care physician appointments on the Cape. My father relied on Marie. He didn't retain information, and he confused instructions.

The primary care physician decided on my father's healthcare based on Marie's beliefs, opinions, and narrative of me. When I looked at my father's medical records, I discovered that the primary care physician noted *family tension. The daughter is power of attorney and health care proxy. She does not agree with the treatment course for father and wife.* But my father's medical decisions were his. Marie and my father did not make joint medical care decisions. And the physician, without discussing it with me or the three of us together, made an opinion solely based on what Marie told her. The physician formed an opinion and a belief based on partial information.

My father's condition continued to deteriorate throughout July 2018. The in-home nurse recommended that Marie take my father to the primary care physician because of his increased wheezing and chronic cough. I received no communication again. Ten weeks before my father's death, the primary care doctor called to make an appointment for a pulmonologist.

My father was supposed to be on palliative/comfort care. Palliative care physicians are specially trained *to prevent and ease suffering for people like my father who need end-of-life care.* I couldn't understand why the primary care doctor took it upon herself to make the appointment, especially because the pulmonologist wasn't considered a palliative care physician.

It was my duty to carry out my father's medical decisions as he wanted. He had been back and forth to the doctor's office multiple times per week, including emergency room visits. My father's symptoms were out of control. I wanted palliative care to begin before hospice to ensure a seamless transition and a coordinated, consistent, continuum of care. I wanted to do everything I could, to prevent unnecessary pain and to ensure at the end of my father's life he would die in comfort.

LESSONS LEARNED

- I learned that an advocate can be a powerful voice, but only when a physician honors those rights.
- The parameters that fall under a physician's beliefs, opinions, morals, values, religion, and ethics are broad and subjective.
- Civil rights guarantee our protection regardless of race, religion, or physical or mental disability.
- Healthcare advocates protect your person. Be present at appointments, monitor medications, and follow up with those who administer them.
- Marie deliberately and willfully cut my father's dosage of memantine in half

My father relied solely on Marie, who was his caretaker, to give him his medications. The medication she cut in half prevented my father from having the full benefit of memantine. Studies have shown that this drug increases memory, awareness, and concentration. This drug might have allowed him to recall a memory, what was happening at the moment, and to calm the agitation he felt after sundown. But Marie willfully deprived him of the full dosage, lowering his chances of it ever happening.

"Willful deprivation is a type of elder abuse. It means denying an older adult medication, medical care, shelter, food, a therapeutic device, or other physical assistance, and exposing that person to the risk of physical, mental, or emotional harm—except when the older, competent adult has expressed a desire to go without such care."[34] From the National Council on Aging, "Get the Facts on Elder Abuse."

Chapter 18

The Quest for Guardianship

Marie had skillfully placed me in the category of *not to be trusted*. Her ambition, when my father was nearing the end of his life, was to embark on a court battle. She wanted guardianship and she dug in, grabbed on, and didn't let go of her desire to tear my father apart from me and my brother. Looking back, I can say with certainty I should have had a social worker as part of my father's care team from the moment of my father's Alzheimer's diagnosis.

My mind was going a million miles a minute. Why did Marie tell the primary care physician I did not agree with what she and my father wanted for treatment? On June 20, 2018, I called patient advocacy. I wanted to fix the lack of communication issue with the primary care physician. The patient advocate informed me Marie had been meeting with a social worker.

I said, "That's good. But I'd like her name and contact number because I want to meet with her and share my side of the story."

Besides a one-on-one meeting, I requested the social worker to conduct mediation with myself and Marie. And what better person than the social worker who already had a background on Marie and our family?

The social worker could meet. For a solid hour, I showed irrefutable evidence that Marie had continually blocked me from receiving my father's medical information. I showed her the emails I sent to the doctor when we stopped chemo as a family, followed by the pages of my father's medical chart, living will, and healthcare proxy. I wanted her to see the truth. Marie said to my father's primary care physician, that I went against my father's wishes. And she believed Marie. But it wasn't true, and the social worker listened. She read the documents that I highlighted.

I said, "I am being prevented from doing what my father appointed me to do."

Since all this madness began, the social worker was the first person I talked to who heard what I was saying. After she reviewed the documents and physician's notes, she agreed.

She said, "I hear you and I have to tell you that Marie has painted a totally different picture."

I met the social worker at Marie's the following day for mediation. My brother offered to pick up my father for lunch while Marie and I had our meeting. The social worker played a critical role in getting Marie to accept me as my father's advocate. She acknowledged my father gave me permission to speak for him and act for him on his behalf. The social worker made it clear to Marie that I could move my father, but it wasn't what I wanted to do. I wanted to honor my father's wishes and allow him to stay in his home.

The social worker said, "If you go to court Marie, you will not win."

The social worker made Marie accountable for her actions. After some deliberation, Marie agreed to communicate with me about my father's health. But then she sat back in the armchair and crossed her arms on top of the kitchen table and cocked her head to the side.

Marie said, "So, you want me to call you even if he has a cold?"

I replied, "Yes."

Marie belittled and minimized my concerns. This is what it was like with her. It was constant and exhausting. But finally, I thought, *I can stop defending myself.* I had someone who believed me and saw Marie. The social worker was monumental in regaining my father's voice.

The social worker said, "Marie, Jacqueline, you have known each other for twenty years. You are family."

We shook our heads in agreement.

She said, "I know there is love there."

Marie's body language softened, and she lowered her guard. We hugged, and it seemed we had agreed. I thought for sure that from now on, we would be on a much more even keel. I felt relieved. I thought this was the turning point.

I never thought about what going to court meant, and I bypassed it. It wasn't until four years after my father's death while writing this book that I reached out to the same social worker. She confirmed Marie had been pursuing legal guardianship. Marie wanted to remove me as my father's advocate for no legitimate reason, other than, she wanted total control over my father's medical decisions, his finances, and all his assets.

Marie wasn't granted guardianship. And in three months before my father died, Marie couldn't just let us just *BE* with my father. She tried, with all her might, to eradicate me and my brother, and in her pursuit, she destroyed the peace my father deserved.

⸺⸺⸺

On June 21, 2018, I called the radiologist for my father. I begged them for a referral for hospice. My father had been on a nonstop merry-go-round of doctor's visits. Before the close of the business day, the secretary called me back and granted hospice for my father. Communication with Marie was going well. It had been two weeks and there were no major issues, but in mid-July, I got a call from Marie's phone. She had passed the phone to the paramedic from the local fire department to speak to me first. They were at home. My father had collapsed on the bathroom floor, and Marie couldn't get him up. The paramedic passed the phone back to Marie.

She said, "You wanted me to call you, so I'm calling."

I asked, "What happened?"

She said, "I gave him morphine and he collapsed. He's being transported to Falmouth Hospital."

I said, "Okay, Mark and I are on our way. We're in Worcester now."

We started driving toward the highway before I hung up the phone. We arrived at the hospital two hours later. I saw my father in the curtained partition in the emergency room as Mark and I were walking down the hallway. He was lying on the gurney with his eyes closed and his feet hanging out from under the sheet. He was in rough shape.

Marie sat beside him in a chair, reading a magazine. We asked her if the doctor had updated her on his condition, but he hadn't yet. I heard him wheezing from where I stood. He wore an oxygen mask, and his face was ashen white. His chest echoed as he coughed, and he choked from the build-up in his lungs. I fixed the blankets on his bed and covered his feet, then soaked a washcloth with cool water and rang it out to put on his forehead. There was no relief for him. We were there for hours while they stabilized him.

We had been there about six hours before his condition improved and we needed to wait for his release before he could go home. The nurse said we could drive him, but my husband and I said no way. My father's lungs were failing. We didn't want to risk him having difficulty breathing while we were driving. It was something we didn't want to chance.

We asked if they had medical transport available, which they did, but they told us it might take hours if that's what we wanted to do. Marie wanted to drive him, but we explained to her it was better for him if we waited.

The transport arrived about 8 pm, the drive home took half an hour and by 9 pm he was in his bed. He seemed ok when they left. But within an hour, he broke out in a coughing fit again. He was choking and struggling to inhale to catch his breath just as he was in the hospital. We propped him up with pillows and put the humidifier on with eucalyptus next to his head. When that didn't seem to do anything, we had him lean over. I cupped my hand and firmly patted his back, dislodging the mucus that clogged his lungs. He hacked and coughed, but nothing came up or out. He urgently needed help.

I called the hospice nurse. She arrived about midnight. My father had to go to the bathroom, but he couldn't stand or put one foot in front of the other, even with our help. He was too weak.

I was in the kitchen with Mark while the nurse tried to put in a catheter. He screamed, and she tried a few times and with each scream, we doubted the hospital's decision for him to come home. We didn't know if he should go back. The nurse wanted to try one more time, but we were already thinking, *what do we do next if we can't get him stabilized?* Finally, she did, and my father fell asleep. I told Marie that Mark and I were going home, and I'd be back in a few hours.

The next morning, my husband and I arrived at my father's house on the Cape. The visiting nurse was there, and my father was sitting in the kitchen. My brother got there before us. He carried my father's recliner from upstairs to the downstairs bedroom off the kitchen. When my father stood from the table to move into the bedroom, he couldn't. My brother and Mark tried to stand him up and guide him, but he wobbled and had no strength at all in his legs. We didn't want him to fall. The last thing he needed was a broken hip. We suggested the nurse call the fire department for a lift assist.

My father felt embarrassed and when the fire department arrived, he apologized to them for having to come out. We informed the firefighters he had retired from Boston Fire. The guys talked with him as they moved him. They asked him about his time on the job and the whereabouts of Ladder 7 in Boston. They made him feel valued. He was their fellow brother, and they returned to him his dignity and they were genuine.

When they left, I told the visiting nurse I didn't want to leave him at home alone with Marie. I asked the visiting nurse if we could place him in a short-term facility until I figured out what to do because he needed more supervision. Marie opposed the idea. She wanted my father to stay at home with her. Marie tried to reassure me. She said she'd call me if something happened. I didn't see how it was possible. My father needed more care. He was a fall risk, and his symptoms were not under control by any means. He needed to be monitored.

The nurse felt for Marie and supported her. But their home wasn't the best place for him under the circumstances. The short-term facilities in the area were full. There was another facility that had an open bed, but the nurse said you don't want to go there. We were scrambling. We couldn't admit him into the hospital, and I didn't have 24-hour care set up. The nurse kept trying, and a bed became available in Falmouth later that afternoon.

My brother and I followed the transport and stayed a while before going home. The next morning, the nurse on duty called me and said my father had done a 180. He was alert, pacing the floors and he wanted out. I drove down and signed the discharge papers. Marie was already there by the time I arrived. They released my father, and Marie took him home. I drove home thinking, *now what?*

When I got home, I talked with Mark, and I told him I wasn't sure how to manage this. If I called a memory care facility to admit him, the chances are they'd have a waitlist. We couldn't wait. Without hesitation, Mark jumped in and said bring him here with us. I called Marie and explained that we wanted to move my father in with us. I said, "I can't do it anymore. I can't manage his care from two hours away. Dad is failing and he needs more care. You are welcome to stay at our house. Mark and I are setting up a private room on the first floor. You can come and go as you please. Dad's care will be done from home." The visiting nurse who was checking in on my father got on the phone and said my father was stable and doing well.

She said, "I see no reason your father shouldn't stay home with Marie."

I could hear the empathy she had for Marie in her voice. She tried to persuade me to leave him at home.

I said, "No, I can't do it. I've made up my mind. He's coming home with me and Mark."

I had made up my mind and no one could change it.

LESSONS LEARNED

- **I suggest advocates research** short-term and long-term care.
- Visit Medicare.gov to find and compare nursing homes, hospitals & other providers near you.
- Compare multiple providers, their quality ratings, and services.
- Sometimes, in an emergency, choices are limited to the center with an open bed. These can range from excellent to good, fair and poor.

Chapter 19
Hospice:
Their Mission vs. Their Capability

The mission to offer comfort and peace at the end of one's life journey is a core principle of hospice dating back to the 1800s. Hospices pledge to treat patients with dignity. They offer physical, emotional, and spiritual support to those who are dying and their families. Pain management is their primary goal. It is their job.

It became difficult to discern from a hospice webpage, who had the care that best fit the needs of my father. I read several mission statements. All the hospices highlighted their commitment and ability to provide pain relief and emotional and spiritual support for the individual and the family. Comfort meant being free from pain, but what I learned was that not every hospice delivers the promises they make.

My go-to method of deciphering good from bad, back then, was to ask people I knew and trusted. In this instance, I asked my husband because he had lived in the Worcester area for most of his life and he worked in the city as a firefighter. He made a few calls. A couple of friends recommended a hospice in Worcester.

The hospice website showed their hospice house in Worcester. It sat almost hidden in a residential neighborhood on a cul-de-sac. Flowers and trees filled the landscape, flowing down and around the pond in the back, providing a view from each patient's room. The hospice stated its goals and values. Their mission statement caught my attention, especially their commitment to tailoring care to the patient's individual needs. It prompted me to call and schedule an appointment to visit the hospice and learn more.

Fear Knocked — Jacqueline Sullivan Wyco

It was late summer. The exact time of year my mother died. I was twenty-six years old then. Now, at fifty-three, that same feeling of disbelief surrounded me. It hit me as soon as I walked up the pathway to the hospice entrance. I didn't want to be there. It made me nauseous.

Mark rang the doorbell, and they let us in and said the director would be with us shortly. I scanned the place as we were waiting. The entryway opened into a main area with vaulted ceilings with a view of the second-floor lounge area. A few people up there were quietly talking. There were snacks, coffee, and a kitchen area off to the side. A large sliding glass door led out to a deck overlooking the trees, flowers, and the pond. It felt peaceful. It was quiet and serene. So far, in a brief couple of minutes, we saw no signs of concern.

When the director came over, she gave us an overview of the layout from where we stood. On the right side of the building were patients' rooms. They were all private, located both upstairs and downstairs. She showed us a couple of rooms to get an idea of what to expect if my father had to be admitted. Each room overlooked the pond. It appeared exactly as depicted on their website. She explained the purpose of the hospice house.

The director said, "When pain becomes unmanageable, they come here and whether it was at home, in a nursing home, or any other facility where they live, patients can come here and get their pain under control."

On our way out, Mark and I noticed a man sitting in the hallway, next to the door. We asked him if he had a loved one staying there. He said his wife was dying. We told him we were sorry, and that we were taking a tour in case we needed to come here. He said in his opinion, the care his wife received was good. With all the information I had, I transferred my father's care to the hospice on August 7, 2018. I felt reassured of my decision because the hospice house was there for us in case we could not manage my father's pain at home.

Mark and I got my father's room ready at our house. Marie drove him the next day. Mark brought home an adjustable bed, and every item to make my father feel comfortable and Marie welcomed.

We wanted peace for my father. It had been an ongoing struggle with the primary care physician and Marie's constant efforts to obstruct me from being my father's legal advocate. At this time, we didn't know he had thirty-seven days of his life left. I knew how incredibly fortunate we were to be near him these last days. I felt more at ease now, knowing he was going to be with us.

The day after my father and Marie arrived, the hospice nurse manager visited to conduct the in-home evaluation. We sat at the kitchen table, and I asked the nurse to speak to us without my father first. My father forgot he had Alzheimer's and lung cancer. In his mind, he wasn't dying. The hospice placed priority on ensuring freedom from pain, and the nurse explained to us anxiety is pain and from a medical standpoint they would treat it as such.

The nurse explained in her introduction hospice would not be there every day. They'd begin at one or two days a week. My husband and I emphasized to her that our priority was to keep my father free from pain and to make his transition from life to death comfortable.

The nurse manager pledged: "This is what we do. The hospice house is there for you. For respite, if you need a break, and if or when your father's pain becomes unmanageable at home. There they can administer drugs for pain that you can't give at home. We have an interdisciplinary care team approach. All team members, including the hospice physician, meet once a week. We discuss patients, who are having difficulties, and we problem-solve as a team."

I was positive I had made the right choice. I felt secure in the plan, and I was confident that my father would die in comfort and in peace.

The social worker made her visit separately.

The social worker said, "Hospice is here for you and your family, so you can concentrate on being a family. My job is to support your father, you, and your family. I am here for you anytime you need me. I am only a phone call away."

My husband stayed home with my father, during the two to three days I worked. He cooked his meals and gave him his shower, and meds. He made sure he was comfortable and content. Mark and my father got along great. But I didn't want Mark to have to take on the caretaker role. It takes a physical, mental, and emotional toll. Mark cared for his daughter and both his parents before they died. I wanted us to have what the hospice promised they could deliver, which was the peace and comfort my father needed and to allow us to concentrate on being a family.

But the reality was hospice wasn't enough, and the schedule of the nursing assistants didn't fit in with the days and times we needed extra help. And volunteers, again, weren't available, just like at his home on the Cape. I researched private care companies and hired aides to fill in for a few hours on the days I went to work. My father was unsteady on his feet and, most of the time, an aide mostly shadowed him. There wasn't a lot for them to do, really, but I wasn't sure how to adjust and make it all work. We figured it out as we went along.

The nurses were our support system. They were kind and professional. They addressed every concern I had while visiting my father. If medications weren't working, they called the hospice doctor directly when they were at my home. However, managing symptoms was our primary responsibility. It wasn't what I expected hospice to be. It was nerve-racking. I'm not a nurse. I had zero knowledge of managing medication for a person dying with two terminal diseases. Both of which needed different symptom management. Mark and I watched my father constantly gauging when anxiety was in fact anxiety and if we needed to give him medication.

It was hard to tell sometimes with Alzheimer's. Irritability surfaced frequently. We didn't know how to manage it in the beginning. For one thing, we weren't sure if my father was in physical pain and he couldn't communicate it to us, or if his irritability was related to the terminal agitation. We were unsure and became more afraid of his symptoms escalating if we didn't address them right away. As a result, the 24-hour nurse hotline became our lifeline. As days passed, my father's physical pain worsened. His lungs filled with fluid. And his breathing grew more labored, even with the oxygen. We barely had a handle on the anxiety, agitation, and restlessness that occurred during the day. And when the sun went down, it triggered massive confusion. We had the baby monitor set up in my father's room and as soon as we heard him moving around downstairs from our bedroom, Mark got up and helped him settle down. Some nights Mark slept on the couch next to my father's bedroom because he got up so many times.

My father became hyper-obsessive. He intently focused and

became frantic when looking for his wallet or other item. Then there were nights he woke up and forgot where he was. I can't fully explain what it was like to see my father moving through these last stages of life with Alzheimer's. At 79 years old, my father was dying of lung cancer and Alzheimer's. I felt guilty. I couldn't control his meds, his confusion, or anything at this point. I wanted to help him, but I couldn't.

There was a learning curve. Medications didn't always work to manage my father's pain and anxiety, as they should have. Out of sheer frustration, I asked the nurse how long before the medication took effect. Finding the right dosage of medication to relieve pain, anxiety, agitation, and restlessness was like walking on a tightrope. Over the phone, the nurse expressed concern that too much of the medication could worsen the symptoms we were trying to relieve. As a result, there were many days and nights my father struggled. He didn't voice his pain, but you saw and heard how much he was suffering. The secretions in his lungs increased. He sounded as if he were drowning in his own body. There were meds to dry out the secretions, but the nurse said it was best if we waited until he was closer to the end.

It was a constant balancing act, and, on some nights, we were at our wits' end. We had called the nurse hotline so many times that I had to make a chart.

1st Column: —Time of initial call to the 24-hour nurses hotline.

2nd Column: —The name of the medication.

3rd Column: —Dosage amount.

4th Column: —Call back time, if medication didn't begin working in the time frame I was told.

We recorded this information so that when the nurses came, we gave them an accurate account of what we gave him to manage his pain. It wasn't as straightforward as the hospice made it sound in their introduction. It felt more like my father got caught in a riptide. No matter how hard we tried, we couldn't grab hold of him. The harder we tried to manage his pain, the further it got out of control.

LESSONS LEARNED

- "The degree of cognitive decline in a patient with Alzheimer's can be directly correlated with the severity of pain experienced." From Mayo Clinic Health System,[35] "Dementia-Related Pain Management."

- "Many patients receive inadequate pain treatment due to lack of recognition. Patients may have lost the cognitive ability to tell caregivers they have pain with phrases such as this hurts or I am in pain."[36] From Mayo Clinic Health System, "Dementia-Related Pain Management."

- "People with moderate to severe Alzheimer's aren't able to express or rate their pain on a scale of 1 to 10."[37] From Mayo Clinic Health System, "Dementia-Related Pain Management."

- "The Pain Assessment in Advanced Dementia Scale (PAINAD) was developed to assess pain and reduce the likelihood that it is unrecognized and untreated."[38] From Mayo Clinic Health System, "Dementia-Related Pain Management."

- "It's easy to learn and use by people without prior medical training and does not require the patient to have language skills."[39] From Mayo Clinic Health System, "Dementia-Related Pain Management."

Chapter 20
The Struggle to Maintain Peace

Is it possible to genuinely love a person and despise them at the same time? I learned more about Marie in these past months than I had in twenty years. Since my father married Marie in 2013, she had said, *love you* to me every time before I hung up the phone with my father. I responded, *love you guys*. Our feelings were mutual. But when I took over my father's finances and became involved in his medical decisions, Marie's feelings toward me changed. She despised me. And it was unquestionable.

    Realistically, Marie's feelings towards me could have been related to a stress response, as a caretaker for my father. His Alzheimer's, cancer, and imminent death were a lot for her to face. However, Marie's hostility grew when I acted and spoke on behalf of my father, as he intended. It didn't matter that we were family, and we loved each other. Marie retaliated when I got in the way of her plans. And when Mark offered to bring my father home with us and stepped in to help care for him during hospice, she turned on him too.

    Marie stayed with Mark and me with my father, from Thursday late afternoon to Sunday. She went home to the Cape for the rest of the week. While she stayed with us, she liked to take my father out for a coffee, or lunch. They would be gone for three or four hours and when they arrived home to our house, my father couldn't hold himself up. Mark and I had to steady him from the car across the driveway. He clutched onto our shoulders like a pair of crutches and his legs wobbled beneath him as we sandwiched him between us. By the time we reached the stairs, it was all he could do to stand up, never mind climbing the one and half flights.

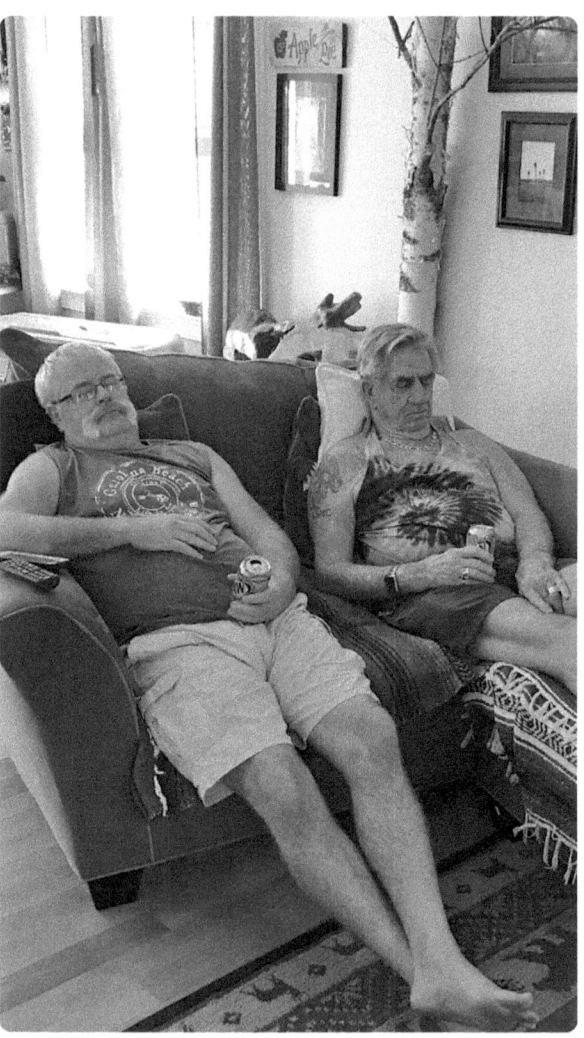

Jacqueline's husband Mark and her father fell asleep watching TV - taken at the author's home on August 27, 2018 -- 17 days before her father died.
Photo by Jacquiline Sullivan Wyco

I called for portable bottles of oxygen for future rides with Marie. Mark and I thought it would help him. But even with the oxygen, it became too much for my father. His lungs had been filling with fluid. The tumor had grown, and the cancer spread. My father grew weaker by the day. His body called for more rest and physical exertion made him bedridden. It became a predictable cycle. And it took a toll on my father. When Marie left for her three days, my father spent the next two to three days in bed. And by the time Marie returned the following week, my father had recovered. With rest, my father sat up with us in the living room and ate a meal in the kitchen. He watched the Red Sox, sipped his tea, and just enjoyed being with us.

I called the social worker assigned to my father's case and asked if she could come out and talk with Marie. I explained my father's extreme weakness and fatigue after he went out with Marie for those three to four-hour periods. I didn't want to engage with Marie over this. Things had finally mellowed out with her. Marie would have taken it as a confrontation coming from me.

The social worker said, "I live thirty minutes away. I think you can do this on your own. You don't need me to do this. Can't you handle it?"

The social worker had done a complete turnaround. She went from being there for our family anytime, day or night, to removing herself completely. Marie did not view what my father needed as a priority. Her needs overshadowed his. This wasn't new. What Marie wanted came first and when she didn't get it, she came at us and inflicted wounds that no one else saw or believed possible. Alzheimer's made my father the perfect victim. And the feeling of being left alone to manage this situation with Marie fried my nerves.

I had to go to work for a few hours. I sat in my car in the driveway, thinking it would be a relatively quick call. I never expected the social worker's reluctance. I thought, *why did she commit herself to our family if thirty minutes was too far to drive for her?* She assured us, as part of the hospice team, that she would be there for us. She was aware of the recent history with Marie, and her attempts to block me and my brother from my father's life. Alzheimer's made my father the perfect victim. But the social worker for whatever reason distanced herself.

I said, "You told me you were here for us so we could concentrate on being a family. I need your help. I can't do this. I cannot talk to Marie without you. I know this from experience. I need your help. Can you please come out and talk with her? I can't do it."

The social worker thought about it. She didn't say yes right away. Finally, after a few minutes, she said, "Okay, I'll come out."

I felt relieved the social worker spoke with Marie, and I didn't have to. But the peace in our family was short-lived. A couple of days later, I got a call from Mark on my way home from work later that Friday afternoon, at about 5 pm.

Mark said, "I can't do it. I can't take it. I'm on my way to get a beer."

I knew whatever happened must have been bad. It took a lot for Mark to get undone. It wasn't like him escaping to a bar for a drink when something bothered him.

I said, "What happened? What's going on?"

Mark said, "Marie was sitting next to your father when I went to give him his meds."

Marie said, "We were all set to go out to eat, but now we can't because Jack's too tired from the medicine."

Mark said, "I reminded your father that he had cancer. And I gave him medicine to help him. Then I said to Marie, *Jack is tired from lung cancer, not the medicine.*"

Mark said, "Your father got angry. *What cancer*, he said. *I don't have cancer.*"

I asked, "Where was Marie?"

Mark said, "She sat beside your father and said nothing."

Mark said, "Later when I went to give your father his med again, he said to me, *WHAT'S THAT?* He snarled at me. He looked like he wanted to kill me. Then Marie turned to me and said, "It's okay. I'll take care of it." Then she took the medicine and your father out on the porch with her."

That's when Mark needed to leave. Yes, my father's reaction could have happened without Marie's comment or presence, and yes, it could have been agitation and anger related solely to Alzheimer's, but again, I look at Marie and her response. When my father switched from accepting the medication from Mark to viewing Mark as if he were a threat, Marie sat next to my father, without saying a word. She stayed silent. She didn't step in to calm him, or to remind him that the medication Mark had been giving him was used to help him. No, instead, she used the situation to make a power play.

In the past, there had been two separate occasions when the visiting nurses went over my father's medications with Marie in their home on the Cape. Both nurses had explained to Marie that she needed to give my father the full dosage of memantine, which was used to enhance his memory. Marie understood the dosage amount. She said she knew what it was and told them she only gave it to him once a day, not two times as prescribed. That image flashed before me, and I never again assumed Marie followed any type of medical direction. She did not want my father's memory enhanced. If she did, she'd have given him his full dosage. The pain medication Mark gave my father prevented Marie from doing what she wanted. I can't say with certainty she gave him his medication.

Marie was angry because she wanted to go out to eat. Marie repeatedly expressed her anger towards us by igniting it in my father and directing it towards us. This time, she aimed it at Mark. She showed us how easy it was for her to influence my father to react by following her lead. Mark loved my father. And Marie crushed him. She knew how to hurt us. I felt so bad. He and my father didn't deserve it.

When I got home, I went upstairs to compose myself. There was so much I wanted to say to her. Honestly, I was on the brink. I wanted her to understand how I felt. Marie intentionally turned peace into chaos. And I wanted to know why. I came downstairs and told Marie I wanted to talk with her about what happened while I was at work. My father was sleeping in his room. His aide sat on the couch adjacent to Marie on the loveseat. I sat down on the coffee table, facing Marie. Every ounce of energy in me turned hot and flowed to the surface of my skin. I measured my words, and I kept my voice down.

I said, "Why did you tell Dad that the medications made him tired?"

Marie said, "It's true, and I wanted to go out to eat and when he took the medicine, he was too tired to go out."

I said, "This isn't about you, Marie, and what you want. This is about Dad, and he is dying. Mark didn't deserve to be treated like that."

Marie grew dismissive. Then she cut me off.

She said, "Okay, you've made your point."

My father was dying, and when she didn't get what she wanted, she made others suffer. I remembered the social worker on the Cape who met with me to speak to Marie about communicating with me. She was firm and direct with Marie. With no emotion, the social worker placed accountability back onto Marie by setting the expectation with a boundary and a consequence for crossing it. Marie's choice became to honor the boundary or cross it and expect a consequence.

I couldn't take it anymore. I wanted her to stop. I had to get through to her and leave my anger toward what she had done out of it.

I leaned forward and locked my eyes on hers.

I said, "Marie, if you ever try anything like that again, I will ask you to leave, and you will not be welcomed back."

And I got up and walked away. This was insanity.

LESSONS LEARNED

I cannot express how sorry I am that I didn't step in sooner to advocate for my father and remove him from Marie's influence. I assumed Marie's actions were related to the stress and anxiety of my father's illness. I thought Marie felt like she was entitled to say or do anything because of her commitment to my father. I didn't link her actions to anything else. "To assume harm and abuse is the consequence of the stressful demands of caregiving minimizes accountability on the part of the perpetrator and fails to consider the criminal nature of the behavior. Coercive and controlling behavior often also remain undetected.[40] "From The Conversation, "The Combination of Dementia and Domestic Abuse Is All Too Often Overlooked."

Chapter 21
Nearing The End

Imagine the protective sheathing of every nerve, every single solitary fiber of your mind and body scraped away. You are literally one giant raw nerve, on edge 24/7, seven days a week, with no reprieve. Then, with a wave of clarity, a sudden rush of euphoria washes over you. But the realization of death sets in with a profound sadness that you have never experienced before. And the visions. No one can see them other than you. What I have described is the terminal agitation my father became afflicted with during the last two weeks of his life.

My father called me from downstairs at one in the morning, not knowing where he was. When I entered his room, he turned strangely euphoric. My father was caught between two worlds. He had to let go of this life to move on to what came next for him.

He said, "Well, at least it's a short trip. The roads are really nice. I'm going downstairs to wait in line to get my hand stamped. Jacqueline, where am I again?"

I said, "You're at my house, Dad."

He said, "Oh, wow, this place is yours? What a place. I'm so proud of you, and John. You are the two greatest kids. I just want to tell everyone. And you're married, right? To Mark?"

"Yes, Dad."

He said, "Oh, he's a nice guy. I feel safe with him."

Feeling safe triggered him. It unnerved me to think that he ever felt unsafe. I noticed with his Alzheimer's that there were moments of clarity in which he expressed what he experienced. And I wondered why he never said anything before. I found this advice: "With coercive

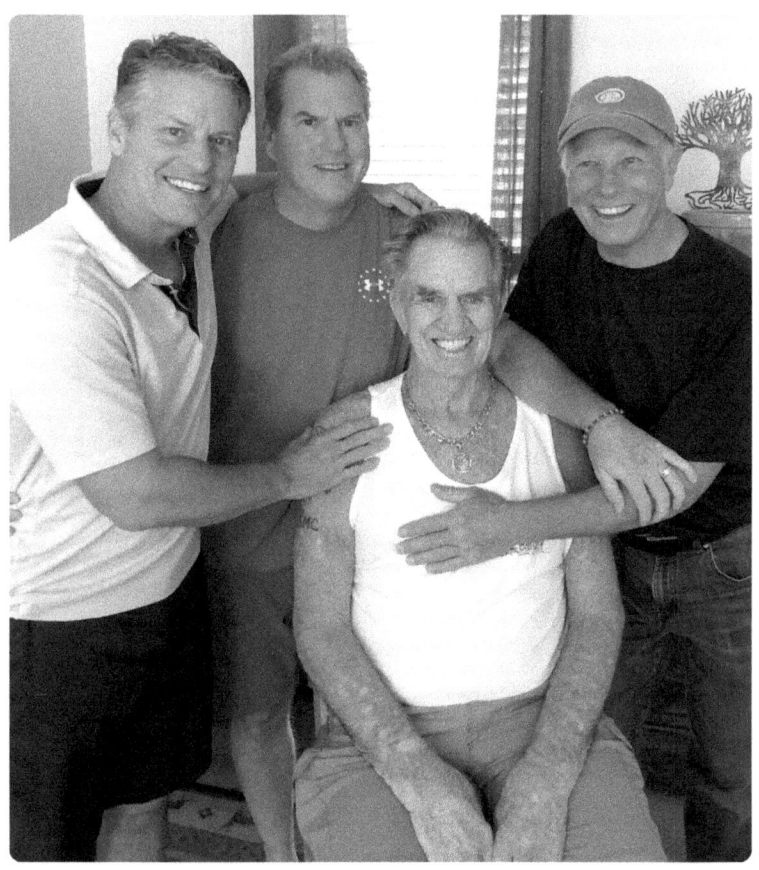

Final farewell to great friends, California firefighters John (Jack) met on the Big Ride. From left to right, Joe Novelli, Mike Keefe, John, and George Piscitello. 13 days before John's death. *Photos by Jacqueline Sullivan Wyco*

control in particular, the older person might be told if they speak out they will be punished—sent to an aged care home or not allowed visitors."[41] From Compass Guiding Action On Elder Abuse, "Understanding Coercive Control as Elder Abuse."

I questioned myself why I didn't move him sooner. My father had confirmed to me we had done the right thing by bringing him home to be with us.

My father was on an intense high. I tried to get him to relax, and I talked to him.

"It's late, Dad. You need to try and sleep."

I got him to lie down and pulled his comforter up over his shoulder. The night light was just bright enough to where I could see his face. I sat in the recliner at the end of the bed and watched him until he closed his eyes. Thoughts of life without him ran through my head as he nodded off. I hoped he could rest for a while. But the reality was we weren't managing my father's terminal agitation and pain. We were chasing it. His symptoms were spiraling out of control.

When the nurse came the next morning, she described my father as having terminal agitation. According to her, not everyone experiences this phenomenon. "Terminal restlessness is a particularly distressing form of delirium that sometimes occurs in dying patients. It is characterized by anguish (spiritual, emotional, or physical), restlessness, anxiety, agitation, and cognitive failure. Delirium is common towards the end of life and is a phenomenon that can have different causes. However, sometimes delirium is part of the final stages of dying—so-called terminal delirium or terminal restlessness—and it becomes an irreversible process that is often treated symptomatically, with the goal of providing comfort (i.e., sedation) instead of reversing the syndrome."[42] From Verywell Health, Terminal Restlessness and Delerium at the End of Life.

I believe it was my father's determination, his strength, and his will to live that caused the intense emotional fluctuations and the sudden rushes of euphoria. But, too, I wondered if, on some level, he was aware of every event leading up till now.

In the nurse's opinion, it looked as though my father had only about two weeks left.

Fear Knocked — Jacqueline Sullivan Wyco

She said, "Once a week we have a group meeting with the hospice physician and other nurses, to discuss patient cases. I'm going to bring your father's case up to the In Team to see what they could do other than what we have tried to do so far to manage his pain."

Mark and I said to the nurse, "Our main priority is to keep my father free from pain and comfortable."

The nurse manager said, "We will. Pain management is what we do."

Marie was on her way home to the Cape after the meeting. I asked her while she packed if she would bring one of my father's suits back with her. With only a couple of weeks left, I planned my father's wake and funeral, our last tribute to the man we loved so much. I wanted to spend some time composing his obituary. For my mother, I wrote her eulogy, and I read to her what she meant to us as she lay unconscious in the hospital. For my father, I would read him his obituary while he was asleep. Both my parents fought death until their bodies failed.

My father was exuberant. He loved life and people gravitated towards him. His obituary needed to reflect him, and it had to jump off the page. For those who loved him, I wanted to capture what made him special and for those who were on the obit page just scrolling through, I wanted to snag their interest and hold their attention. The first couple of lines of his obituary filled you in on who he was. *No matter how many times Jack got knocked down, he got up twice as many. Jack fought hard as hell to stay. Alzheimer's and lung cancer couldn't keep Jack from wanting to live.* That was the beginning and by the end, nine hundred and eighty words filled a quarter of a page of the Boston Sunday Globe. https://www.milesfuneralhome.com/obituaries/John-Jack-Sullivan-2/#!/obituary.

Mark suggested that we call my father's friends to say goodbye. I had done it for my mother, but it didn't dawn on me until he brought it up. We called Murray first, my father's partner and friend from the fire department. He was back in Massachusetts for the summer, not too far away from where we lived. When we invited him to come over, he asked if we were sure because he didn't feel that my father wanted to see him. I received a voicemail from him about two weeks prior. He described the hurt he felt by my father's refusal to speak with him. He said that Marie told him Jack didn't want to talk to him. My father somehow thought Murray got a gang of kids to punch him in the stomach down at the pool.

Murray said, "I understand the long goodbye. If I'm a casualty of the disease, I can deal with it. But your father and I have been friends for years and I don't get where this story came from. It bothers me. Where did he get this idea?"

I called Murray after I listened to his voicemail. I reaffirmed how much he meant to us.

Fabrication of stories can result from cognitive decline. I'm not sure why Marie perpetuated this story. During this time, my father had no recall. My father jumbled facts and combined stories, often forgetting the names of his friends and others. As I explained earlier, Marie told me back in Florida that she and my father did not talk to Murray anymore. At first, she didn't know why, then she told me this story later when I asked how Murray was. Then mysteriously the rift blew over. However, now it seemed the rift returned.

Marie molded my father's beliefs in less time than it takes to blink your eyes and if she had told my father they did not talk to Murray anymore because of A, B, C, or D, then he went along with it. My father could have come up with this story and this is not uncommon for people living with Alzheimer's, but that wasn't the issue. Marie told Murray that my father didn't want to speak with him, not my father. It was Marie who alienated Murray.

Let's say I'm wrong. Marie is innocent, and I've pointed my finger where I shouldn't. That still wouldn't explain why Marie reinforced my father's loss of trust in Murray as a friend. If that story came from my father, it was a figment of a delusion related to his disease. Murray was a great friend and confidant. That never changed. But Marie fostered this separation between him and my father. She controlled the narrative. And attached the blame to my father, not his disease.

Mark assured Murray that my father wanted to see him. My brother came out the same day too. Marie wasn't there, and we planned it that way. Her absence allowed us time to sit back, relax, and speak without her hanging over my father's every word. When Murray and my father talked, it was like old times. My father treasured their relationship. There was no doubt Marie could have bridged the gap in my father's memory and the perceived divide in their friendship. The proof was sitting in my living room. Even if she didn't make my father understand or change his mind, she could have reassured Murray that my father's friendship was important to him and that it was his disease talking, not him. Murray had been the nearest and dearest of friends, and Marie offered him no solace. She could have thanked him for all the years of friendship he had given her and my father, but she didn't. Instead, she stomped on his heart and yanked out his feet from beneath him. She convinced him his friendship with my father was over.

A couple of days passed, and I made our next call to my father's friend Mike, in California. Mike, George, Joe, and my father were like-minded souls who met and became inseparable along the 3,300-mile trek from Seattle, Washington to Washington, DC on the Big Ride. My father loved those guys. They were more like family than friends and when he described them, he said they were the type of guys who would give you the shirt off their back. I called Mike and told him I didn't know if he knew my father had Alzheimer's. He didn't know, and I wished I had told him sooner. When I said he had lung cancer and only had a couple of weeks left, Mike wanted to visit him. But he wondered if my father remembered him. I told him I had no doubt that he did. He called Joe and George. And in less than 24 hours, they pulled into our driveway.

Marie was there that day. She met Mike, George, and Joe with me and my brother the day my father rode into Washington, DC. We got to know them over the years through my father. When they arrived at our house to say farewell, I went into my father's bedroom and touched his shoulder to wake him.

I said, "Dad, Mike's here."

My father said his last name.

I said, "Yes, Dad, he's here. In the kitchen."

His eyes opened wide, and he sat straight up and got out of bed. He didn't forget their friendship. When he walked into the kitchen, he couldn't get over it. As soon as he saw Mike, they hugged like two bears. My brother, Mark, and I saw my father light up. He smiled from ear to ear. He was so happy to see them.

When my father finished the Big Ride, he had his bicycle chain turned into bracelets, and he gave Mike and George one, and they both were wearing them. Their friendship was special. My father looked elated. They laughed and reminisced for hours. Mike called home to his wife and kids; they were on speaker with my father. When they hung up, Mike called riders from the Big Ride, and they all talked some more. My kitchen filled with my father's laugh and Marie turned on the charm. She was pleasant and sociable, more like the Marie I used to know.

We took group pictures the next day. Mike, George, and Joe smiled and hugged my father. They held it together in front of him, but we all cried when we walked them out to their car. My father and Marie stayed on the porch. We watched as they drove away, beeped the horn, and waved their arms out the window. We waved back until we couldn't see them anymore. As we walked back into the house, we composed ourselves. My father came and sat with us at the kitchen table. It was beyond sad. It was another stark reminder that my father was in his last days. We felt deflated. Marie was busy, bouncing back and forth between the bedroom and the kitchen as she packed her bag. My father asked her where she was going.

Marie said, "Going home."

She had one foot out the door before my father's friends had left the driveway. My father had just said goodbye. While Mark, my brother, and I were sitting with him, he bowed his head and looked down at his hands resting on the table.

My father said, "I'll never see my buddies again."

He was grieving, and now Marie was leaving too. When my father's friends were there, Marie turned on the charm. She was a doting wife and a loving family member. As soon as they left, she shut it down. She wanted out of there. It was Sunday, her day to leave and go home, and the loss my father felt didn't change her plans. He was mourning, and the separation between him and his friends was a final one. He knew in those moments that he was dying, and Marie carried on, packed her bags, and left.

Alzheimer's had forced the separation of who my father was from his memory, and it held him hostage and unjustly punished him with anxiety, restlessness, agitation, delirium, and confusion for years. But this wasn't the worst. Alzheimer's was about to merge with end-of-life pain so violent and agitation so intense and overwhelming that it still brings tears to my eyes.

LESSONS LEARNED
FAQs: Pain Management in Hospice Care
Here are questions about managing pain while in hospice, according to the Continua Group:

What pain meds do they use in hospice?
Hospice care providers use a range of pain medications, including opioids (morphine, hydromorphone, oxycodone), non-opioid analgesics (acetaminophen, NSAIDs), and adjuvant medications (antidepressants, anticonvulsants, corticosteroids).

What pain medication is given at the end of life?
Potent opioids, such as morphine or hydromorphone, are commonly used to manage pain at the end of life due to their effectiveness and ease of titration.

Does hospice focus on pain management?
Pain management is a primary focus of hospice care, as it significantly impacts the patient's quality of life and comfort.

How is pain managed at the end of life?
Pain at the end of life is managed using a combination of pharmacological interventions (opioids, non-opioid analgesics, adjuvant medications) and non-pharmacological approaches (emotional and spiritual support, complementary therapies).

What is the opioid of choice for pain relief at the end of life?
Morphine is often considered the opioid of choice for pain

relief at the end of life due to its efficacy, availability, and ease of titration.

What hospice medication is stronger than morphine?
Hydromorphone and fentanyl are opioids that are more potent than morphine and may be used in certain situations for pain management in hospice care."[43] From Continua Group, "Hospice Pain Management: A Comprehensive Guide."

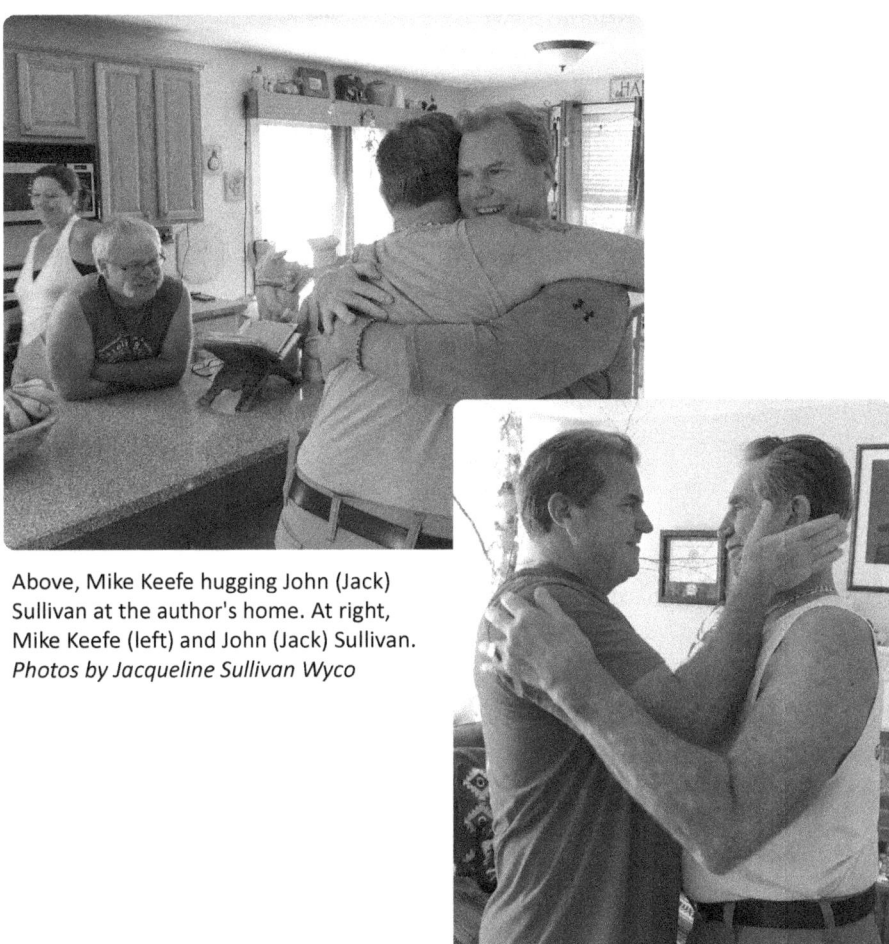

Above, Mike Keefe hugging John (Jack) Sullivan at the author's home. At right, Mike Keefe (left) and John (Jack) Sullivan.
Photos by Jacqueline Sullivan Wyco

Chapter 22

Pain Out of Control

My father pushed himself and lived life beyond his comfort zone. Throughout his life, he set goals and challenged himself. His body went through some grueling feats. His pain tolerance was remarkably high. I witnessed over the years how he used his mind to dull the pain. He reduced pain by removing it from his focus, or as he used to say, by putting it on the back burner. But Alzheimer's had changed that. No longer was he able to will it away, and he lost the ability to describe how it felt. Mark and I noticed clear signals of distress, and the pain medication dosage the hospice instructed to give wasn't aggressive enough to override what was happening in his body. My father was being ravaged physically, mentally, and emotionally from the inside out.

We needed to know what else to try. When the nurse came for her visit, we said we never expected that his pain would be so out of control. There had to be something else to do. She immediately texted the doctor. He was at the office in the team meeting. They were in the middle of discussing my father's case. He suggested admitting him to the hospice house, which we discussed from the beginning as a last resort.

Mark and I said to the nurse, "What else can we try? Is there anything else the doctor can prescribe? If we can get his symptoms under control, he can stay at home with us. And if we can't, we'll know, he needs to be admitted."

The doctor replied to the nurse.

"Try phenobarbital. It can be administered to him immediately. I advise that he be monitored closely due to the potential severity of its side effects."

The hospice physician waited a long time before he started the more aggressive treatment. The best way I can describe his pain-to-relief ratio response is like a firefighter putting out a three-alarm fire with a garden hose. If we hadn't questioned and pursued alternatives, I don't know when the hospice physician might have shifted to a more aggressive pain medication.

It was Thursday afternoon, and the nurse told us that the hospice pharmacy was closing. If she called in the prescription, they'd mail it, but it may not arrive until Monday because of the weekend. That was three days away, and I didn't want my father to wait. He needed relief. The nurse told us she could call it into our local pharmacy. The next day, it would be ready to pick up. Mark and I went to Walgreens in Holden, the next town over from us, to pick it up, but they didn't fill the prescription. They were out. The pharmacist double-checked, and phenobarbital came up on their computer as none in stock.

It was 6:30 in the evening. I don't know if the pharmacy contacted the hospice nurse. And I'm not sure why there was no follow-up or confirmation by the hospice. But the ball got dropped and the communication breakdown had us scrambling.

I called the 24-hour nurse hotline and explained what was happening. While speaking with her, I walked back into Walgreens to ask the pharmacist to call another pharmacy. She called one in Worcester, the next town over, but they were out too.

The nurse said, "I'll call you back in about forty-five minutes. I'm going to make a few calls and see what I can do."

Mark and I waited in a restaurant across the street from the pharmacy. My phone rang about 7:40. The restaurant filled up for dinner while we waited. It was loud and hard to hear the nurse over the phone.

She said, "I found a CVS in Worcester on the border of Auburn, about 25 minutes away. Can you drive there?"

I said, "Yes. Thank you. We can get there, no problem."

The nurse said, "I'll call it in, and if there's anything else you need, don't hesitate to call."

I thanked her again. This was a fiasco and was a sign of what was yet to come.

The next morning, the social worker visited. While we were talking, the nurse arrived and when she had finished her assessment of my father, she sat with us. We were out of options. The phenobarbital didn't relieve my father's pain. He still wasn't comfortable. We knew that hospice house was the inevitable next step. It was time to admit him.

My mind was racing. How do we make this smooth transition? My father didn't remember he was dying, and I somehow had to convince him to get up from bed and transport him in an ambulance to a completely unfamiliar place. The nurse explained we would sedate him before the transport arrived at 7:30 pm. Mark and I reminded her, that medications that would knock me or my husband out, wouldn't come close to sedating my father. She listened and called the physician immediately to convey our concerns. When she hung up with the physician, she explained palliative sedation again and how to prepare my father for transport.

She said, "You are going to give your father two doses of phenobarbital, four hours apart, the second one being at 6:45 pm."

The nurse said, "Your father will be heavily sedated by the time the ambulance arrives."

My heart wasn't in it. And only a few hours left until transport. I wanted so much for this not to be the end. Soon my father would leave us, and never return.

We acted normally around my father for those last hours, and we watched for the ambulance as the time got closer. Marie packed her bag to leave and planned to follow the ambulance to the hospice house. We walked outside to meet the driver when we saw him pull into the driveway. Marie stayed in the house. Mark and I shook his hand and introduced ourselves.

Mark said, "It's a tight squeeze in the hallway outside the bedroom. These stairs are narrow, too. Are you going to be able to manage with a stretcher?"

Mark said, "I can help you."

The one-and-a-half flights of stairs in the front were shallow and steep. We weren't sure how to get my father down and into the ambulance. Even if we helped, there wasn't enough room to maneuver.

The transport driver said, "It's not a problem. We have a chair with straps. We can get him in it and down safely."

I went into my father's room. He was sleeping on his side. I touched his back to wake him while the driver and medic prepared to carry him down into the ambulance. He woke up instantly. Remarkably, he was more alert than I expected. He got confused when I said, "Dad, we need to go to the doctor's so they can check you out. I need to take your gold chain off and your rings." My mother had given him the chain. It was as big and bold as him. I helped him open the lobster claw clasp and said, "I'll put it with your rings and wallet. We can keep them here."

He sat up and wriggled his wedding band from my mother. He never took it off, even after he married Marie. Then he slid his other gold ring over his knuckle. It was incredible. He had enough tranquilizer in him to keel over an elephant, yet he was coherent and able to talk. He asked where he was going several times in between the medic's questions. I felt so guilty. Although I thought I was doing what was best for him, it still didn't feel right, not in the least. I followed him down the stairs. Mark and Marie got ready to leave. They drove separately. I hopped into the back of the ambulance after they secured my father.

It was a thirty-minute drive, and my father looked out the window beside him as he lay strapped onto the stretcher. It was pitch black, there were no streetlights where we lived, and the driver seemed to hit every pothole. I lost my bearings riding in the back of the ambulance and as we got closer to Worcester, the glare from oncoming headlights made it harder for me to see where we were. I felt anxious and I didn't want my father to pick up on it.

My father said, "There's a lot of traffic, Jacqueline."

I said, "It's like that country song, Dad, *Convoy*."

He remembered and he stayed alert throughout the ride. When the medics transferred him to the hospice house, he thanked the guys. That was him, always thankful to the people who helped him. The nurse recommended I save time and ensure a smooth transition into the hospice by admitting him over the phone, which I did earlier that afternoon. I confirmed every piece of information they needed.

I reiterated I was my father's advocate. And I made sure they understood to call me with any questions. We had entered the final stage of my father's life.

LESSONS LEARNED

- Confirm everything. Medication, orders, equipment deliveries, patient transport time.
- Follow up with nurses if the pain is persistent.
- "Pain management is essential from the time of diagnosis and throughout the disease trajectory. The prevalence of inadequately controlled pain occurring in those with serious illnesses remains unacceptably high. And studies reveal there are barriers to adequate pain relief and patients continue to experience uncontrolled pain in the final weeks, days, and hours of their lives."[44] From Pain Management Nursing, "American Society for Pain Management Nursing and Hospice and Palliative Nurses Association Position Statement: Pain Management at the End of Life."

Chapter 23
The Window

On September 7, 2018, I admitted my father into the hospice house in Worcester, Massachusetts, to gain control over his pain in the final stage of his life. The hospice pastor came by and introduced himself to Mark and me while we waited in the hallway for the nurses to get my father settled into his room.

When the pastor left, Mark and I entered my father's room to find he had dozed off. He looked exhausted but comfortable. However, it didn't last long. His pain returned. The nurse gave him more medication and assured us it would work. His room was next to the patient information desk. I felt more at ease knowing he was so close to the nurses' station.

Marie said, "I'm going to stay for the night."

I said, "Okay. Then maybe Mark and I will go home and come back early in the morning."

Marie said, "No rush. I'll wait until you get here before I leave."

Mark and I said goodnight to her and my father. We lived only thirty minutes away. On our way out, I asked the nurses to call me if my father's condition changed during the night. Admissions called me earlier that day and I thought for sure she placed my number in my father's chart since I confirmed with her, I was my father's advocate.

The next morning, I texted Marie to see if she wanted anything. Mark and I stopped on our way in for a coffee. She texted back, *no, your father had his coffee and ate breakfast already. We be happy.* When we got there, my father was awake. His pain seemed under control. Marie was ready to leave when we arrived. She didn't say when she'd be back.

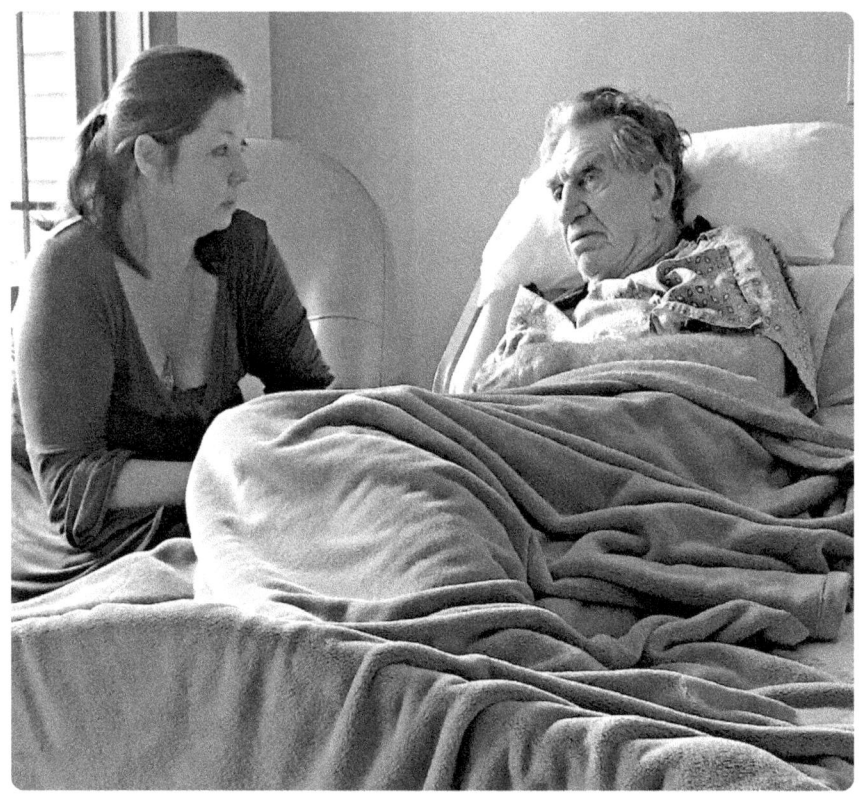

Jacqueline and her father In the hospice home on September 8, 2018. Photo taken by photo taken by John, Jacqueline's brother

My brother arrived shortly after Marie left. Mark was with us in his room when the conversation shifted. He left quietly when he heard my father realize where he was.

My father said, "I know this is it."

"Know what?" my brother said.

My father said, "I know this is it. The end of the line."

"But how?" my brother said.

My father said, "I just know. And it went by so fast."

For the next two hours, my father shared with us his life and what it all meant. He went back to his childhood and reminisced about his parents. When he talked about his mother, he teared up.

He said, "She saved money to buy me the best shoes. We took the train into Boston to the factory. I remember how hard she worked. She had me and my sisters. The four of us. It wasn't easy and she never complained."

Then he went to his dad.

"I miss my dad. Boy, he was a great guy. He never raised his voice. He was a quiet, and gentle man. They called him The Bull, back in Ireland. I'll never forget the story. I had a cousin who lived in the same county. My father rerouted a stream to bring water closer to the house. His mother used to walk quite a way to fill water pails. They had no running water. I don't remember how long it took him, but my father got large boulders and hoisted them up, one on each shoulder. Then he walked through a field and over the top of a hill. He used the boulders to move the direction of the water. And as the sun set behind him, his silhouette appeared to be that of a giant to the people who looked up and saw him from a distance."

My father then picked up his hand and outlined around it in the air.

He said, "His hands were bigger than mine."

Then he shook his head, almost as if he still couldn't believe it.

He said, "He was so strong."

Then he recalled the day his father gave him the money to buy his first car. My father didn't want to take it. He knew his father came here from the old country to work. My grandfather sent most of what he made back home to his mother to provide for his brothers. Then he worked, saved, and sacrificed for his own family.

My father said, "I miss my parents."

Then he retraced the time leading up to his father's death. He sounded coherent. He didn't look like you might imagine a dying man. His voice was strong, and I might have guessed he was much younger if I did not know him. He sat upright as he recounted the blizzard of 1978. He talked as if it had happened yesterday and asked me if I remembered it. The snow was as heavy as cement. My father called it, heart attack snow. The snow cleanup continued for weeks after the storm. My father called my grandfather to tell him he'd be over to plow and shovel. He said, "Dad, I'm headed out to do some more plowing. Don't go out and shovel. It's too heavy. I'll stop up when I'm finished."

His father didn't wait for him. He shoveled. The next morning, just before dawn, my grandmother called our house. My mother answered. My grandfather was having chest pain. My father told her to call 911 and he and my mother jumped in the truck and flew over to their house. They lived only three blocks away.

He said, "I saw it in his eyes as they lifted him into the ambulance. He took one last look around. I knew he wasn't coming back, and he was gone before he reached the hospital."

His father's sudden death knocked the wind out of him. He was devastated when it happened, and I could see it still bothered him. It never sat right with him, because in his mind, if he had gotten up to his father's sooner, he wouldn't have died. My father shook his head and pursed his lips as if in pain.

He said, "If he just didn't go out to shovel."

And that's how his story always ended.

Then he went further back in time again to growing up and the kids on the block he chummed with. He said he wished he hadn't hung around some of them.

"They were kind of trouble. I enlisted because I needed discipline, and I knew the Marine Corps would set me straight."

He stopped for a couple of minutes and stared out the window behind me as if he were gathering his thoughts.

"And Ma, she was unbelievable."

But he couldn't remember her face. I showed him a picture of her, and he studied it.

He said, "She was beautiful. She died so young."

Then he shifted to us.

"I hope I was a good enough father."

I don't know how he could think otherwise, and my brother reminded him.

My brother said, "Dad, you are the best father. You spent so much time with me in baseball, going to my games, and camping every year. I don't know how you did it with working the two jobs. You were always there for us."

We loved him, and we were thankful, and we knew how lucky we were to have him. Not everyone's parents stayed together. And not everyone lived with their father. We knew how much he cared for and loved us, and we made sure he understood how much we appreciated him.

He boasted, "You were the two greatest kids, and you always were."

He seemed to forget some of my teenage years. Towards the end, his last words:

"And love. That's all there is. There's just love. And that's what's important. It all comes down to love."

I tried not to cry, but I couldn't swallow my tears.

My father had just entered a level of consciousness where his soul had connected to the realm beyond his physical being. There was no other explanation, and it was nothing short of miraculous. He didn't want to sit back and rest. He was on a roll and had no intention of stopping.

When the nurse came in to ask him if he wanted lunch, he introduced me and my brother. My father was beaming. He was in that euphoric place again. He ate grilled cheese, chips, and a big bowl of chocolate ice cream. After lunch, I asked him again if he wanted to lie back and close his eyes for a while. I sat by his bed as he stared out the window again.

I said, "I'm going to miss you, Dad. Send us a sign."

You see, the three of us believed in signs. They had connected us to my mother for twenty-six years since her death on the full moon of August 13, 1992. Until then, we had only known the number 13 as an omen, filled with superstition, but after my mother's death, it signified something else. The number 13 appeared to us when we were together and when we were alone. It found its way to us on every special occasion or event, and it appeared out of nowhere, it seemed, when we needed it most. We always knew it was her. Death didn't remove her from our lives, it only changed the way she communicated with us. I wanted that same connection to live on with my father.

My brother kissed my father's forehead and placed his hand between his. We were going to leave for the night and return in the morning. My father's pain was under control.

I didn't know it then, but I realized afterward, it was the window, the space of clarity where he saw the past, present, and future. His life played out in his mind's eye like a reel playing a movie on a screen. It's a phenomenon and not everyone has this experience before death. In a two-hour span, my father reviewed his life and bared his soul. He extracted from his seventy-nine years the pivotal moments, what mattered the most, and he boiled it all down to one word. Love.

LESSONS LEARNED

- Terminal lucidity is the term for what my father experienced. It's a phenomenon.
- "National Institutes of Health study shows surprising activity level in dying brains and may help explain the sudden clarity many people with dementia experience near death. Lucidity was more common than it was the exception in dementia patients, which would suggest that the idea of it being terminal is not entirely correct. Episodes of lucidity should be seen as part of the disease experience rather than as aberrant events. A variety of these episodes occurred months, even years, before the person died, even so, many experts agree that most of these episodes are associated with the approach of death."[45] From Scientific American, "Why Dying People Often Experience a Burst of Lucidity."

Chapter 24
Unfathomable

My father was in a hospice to die in comfort. But it seemed more like he had been blown up in a war zone, buried under a mountain of rubble, trapped and slowly dying for days. His pain was ungodly. My brother and I told my father it was okay to leave. And when he didn't let go, we begged him.

My father's two-hour energy burst depleted him. He wanted to stay awake, but I asked him to close his eyes. His pain was under control. My brother and I thought it was okay to leave. But when I arrived home, a nagging feeling came over me. I wanted to go back.

I said, "Mark, I feel like I should be there."

Mark said, "The nurses will call if anything changes with your father. But if you want, I can drive you back. Whatever you want to do."

I said, "Okay. You're right. I'm going to shower and go to bed."

The next morning Mark stayed home, and I drove to the hospice house for the day. I didn't believe what I saw when I walked into my father's room. I kept my distance as the nurse combed his hair and tucked in his sheets.

They lowered my father's bed to the floor. He sat upright with his eyes closed and his restlessness branched out to every area of his body, including his fingers. He mumbled and swayed like a pendulum while he argued with a person I couldn't see. I took a baby step towards him. Then I froze midway between the door and his bed. I clenched my right hand into a fist against my chest and I squeezed my left hand over it. I didn't go any further.

I asked the nurse, "What happened?"

"He had a rough night. He complained of back pain, and the night nurse couldn't keep him in bed."

My father was unsteady on his feet, a fall risk, and even though the safety rail was up, he got out of his bed. He made it out to the nurses' station before they responded to the alarm attached to him and the bed.

He yelled, "I want to go home. Call me a cab! I want to get out of here!"

That happened two or three times before the nurses had him sit on the couch near them to watch him.

I asked the nurse, "How long do you think he has?"

She said, "Within 24 hours. Would you like me to call the pastor to administer the last rites?"

I said, "Yes."

When she left the room, I sat next to him on the bed and talked to him.

I said softly, "I'm here, Dad."

I called my brother, John.

I said, "I just got here, and it doesn't look good. You better come now."

The pastor came in just as I hung up. He introduced himself again, then placed his hand on top of my father's head and called him John.

"John, you are being called home. Are you tired? Are you ready to return home?"

My father shook his head and mumbled in agreement.

The priest said prayers and offered his condolences to me.

He said, "I'm here if you need me." And he left.

When it was time to reposition my father, I stepped out into the hallway. I went over to the nurses' station and asked the nurse on duty why no one called me the night before when they couldn't keep my father in bed.

I said, "I stopped here last night on my home to make sure I was called if my father's condition changed."

The nurse said, "Marie was called. The nurse put your father on the phone with her and she told him to go back to bed."

Marie was at home on the Cape, two hours away. They didn't

contact me and I couldn't go back to fix it.

I said, "Can you please put my phone number on his chart and on the whiteboard in his room?"

The nurse said, "I'm sorry. Yes, I will."

She didn't understand why I was so upset. *Sorry*, couldn't rewind time when I could have been there for my father. I could have tried to calm him and reassure him. But neither the nurses on duty nor Marie contacted me.

When I returned to my father's room, his pain had increased. When my brother John arrived, my father could no longer verbalize what he needed. Most likely he would be gone in 24 hours. My brother and I weren't leaving. I went out into the hallway and found the laundry closet. I grabbed a couple of blankets and a sheet and laid them beside my father's bed up against the wall. My brother slept in the recliner on the other side. Every four hours, the nurses came in to reposition him, and each time, his pain increased.

24 hours went by. It was now Monday, and his pain was worse. To assess pain in patients who can't communicate, medical staff use observation to detect pain. Non-verbal assessment is based on specific physical observations. My father's chart documented sighs, gasps, moans, groans, and cries. The nurses observed these signs during movement and rest. Their observation included facial grimaces/winces/furrowed brows, narrowed eyes, clenched teeth, tightened lips, jaw drop, and distorted expressions. My father was in acute distress and when pain surged, he grabbed the rail on the bed and squeezed it like he was holding on for dear life. This day when they repositioned him, my brother and I heard him scream from outside in the hallway. It was so loud that it sounded like he was beside us. He yelled, "NO MORE THAT HURTS STOP, THAT'S ENOUGH." He begged them and swore as they moved him.

There was a person at the nurses' station. I wasn't sure who she was, but she wasn't a nurse. I had seen her up in the kitchen area at the coffee station, the day we took a tour.

She said, "I know it's hard, but it's unethical to give too much pain medication in the beginning. It must be given in increments."

Hard didn't describe what we were feeling.

My brother looked at me and said, "They don't let animals suffer like this."

It was brutal. My father's body clenched, and his face showed indescribable pain as he continually moaned and gasped for air. He gurgled so loud, it sounded like someone was holding him down in a lake trying to drown him. The same busybody at the nurses' station told us it was the death rattle. It's not painful. Yes, that is true. If you research death rattle, this is correct. But in hindsight, according to pain observation, if my father had been in comfort, without pain, he would not have been clenching his fists, grimacing in pain, and contracting every muscle in his body. He was, in fact, in pain and discomfort.

We begged my father to die. My brother and I said, "Dad, just let go. Let go."

He wouldn't. I didn't realize he couldn't stretch out in the bed until I noticed him grimacing as he tried to straighten his legs. The bed was too short. He had to keep his legs bent sideways. My brother and I tried using pillows to raise his legs, so his feet might go over the footboard. When that didn't work, I went into the linen closet, got blankets to roll them, and put them under the mattress. It still wasn't high enough for him to stretch out. We then looked to see about removing the footboard, but there weren't any bolts. My father's pain worsened since his admission.

The doctor did not visit all weekend. My father needed pain management and so far, they didn't manage it like we were told. I went to the nurse on duty.

I said, "I want to speak to a supervisor. The person in charge."

The nurse supervisor came down to the basement floor with a social worker. We met in a small room off the waiting area. Both sat next to one another opposite me. I explained to them what my father had been experiencing.

I said, "My father's pain is not being managed. His pain is out of control. And there was a woman who said, it's unethical to give too much pain medication at first."

I said, "She was hanging around at the nurses' station. She wasn't a nurse. I recognized her from up in the kitchen area. Suffering in excruciating pain is part of the dying process, according to her."

I couldn't contain myself. I kept going.

I said, "The bed is too short. He can't straighten out his legs, and when he tries, you can see the pain he is in on his face. My brother and I tried to get the footboard off, but we couldn't."

The nurse supervisor got defensive.

She said, "Most people are happy here."

I said, "I am not most people. His pain needs to be managed."

She said, "His pain is unusual, and it's hard to manage."

I couldn't believe what I was hearing. I sat forward until I was on the edge of the couch.

I said, "He cannot be the first person you have had here in twenty years, that their pain is hard to manage. Pain control is why we are here. We were told by the case manager who met with Dr. Barn, the social worker, and the visiting nurse, that pain management is what the hospice house does. Here, you can use stronger medications that we couldn't give him at home."

The social worker said nothing.

I wanted to scream at the top of my lungs, but I held it in. It should never have come to this, and I don't know why it took this meeting for the nurse manager to make a greater effort to get his pain under control.

Dr. Barn did not visit my father in the hospice home until the fourth day. It was Tuesday, September 11, and I thought my father's suffering would be over. But my father held on. His chest ballooned and filled with air under his left side. He had a fever, and pneumonia and couldn't breathe. His sheets were drenched from his sweat. They were cold and damp. I asked one nurse who came if we could change them. My father wasn't comfortable. He was in pain.

The other nurse on duty played calming music and stroked his head. She comforted him, but the lifting of his body and the repositioning ignited a relentless surge of pain that didn't diminish in intensity for hours at a time. I massaged his legs and feet, but nothing could touch the pain he was in. My father voiced his pain through every excruciating cry. My brother and I didn't know what to do. Marie was at home on the Cape.

It was mid-morning, and I heard a voice in the hallway that I didn't recognize. I went out to see if it might be the doctor. I asked the nurse, and she confirmed it was him. He was working his way down the hallway. At 11:16 am on September 11, 2018, Dr. Barn walked into my father's room with a social worker and a medical student working on her thesis. The two of them stood in the alcove near the door as Dr. Barn walked over to my father in the bed.

Dr. Barn asked me, "Where is your father from?"

I answered, "Boston."

I stood next to my father, who sounded more like a wounded animal than a human. Dr. Barn made small talk. He was indifferent to what was happening. He asked, "Do you have any brothers or sisters?" while my father gasped for air and held on to the bed's side rail as pain surged through his body.

My hand turned white as I gripped the handrail on my father's bed. The doctor's callous attitude made me want to jump over the bed and shake him. We had watched my father suffer for days. We pleaded and begged him to die. Dr. Barn was in no hurry. There was no sense of urgency to medicate my father, to help him breathe more easily, or to free him from the overall torturous pain. We came to the hospice house for end-of-life pain control and pain management. This is what they do. This is what they promised. Dr. Barn's reply to my question, "What are you going to do for him?"

He said, "I am assessing."

Dr. Barn left the room at 11:22 am without saying another word.

I compare Dr. Barn's 6-minute assessment to this. When my father was called to a house fire that was fully involved with civilians trapped, he didn't walk in and make small talk with the people while the fire ate through the walls where they were trapped. My father needed emergency triage, an all-hands-on-deck approach, to assess, strategize, and get his symptoms under control, but that wasn't the case. When Dr. Barn left the room, the nurse stayed.

I said to the nurse, "What's wrong with this doctor? Didn't he see my father? And he's making small talk?"

The nurse looked at me, shook her head from left to right, and rolled her eyes. And said nothing.

LESSONS LEARNED

- Discuss with the hospice an emergency plan of care if they cannot manage pain.
- Agonizing pain SHOULD NOT be endured. Ultimately, if they can't control or manage pain find another hospice.

    "The American Society for Pain Management Nursing and Hospice and Palliative Nurses Association endorse the position that all nurses and other healthcare professionals must advocate for effective, efficient, and safe pain and symptom management to alleviate suffering at end-of-life."[46]

    "To overcome existing obstacles and achieve humane, dignified pain care at the end of life, the following are recommended."

    — "Awareness. In particular, the patient who is nonverbal during the dying process."

    — "Recognition of the need for different routes of medication administration during the dying process."

    —"Accountability of all healthcare professionals to support the patient's and family's wishes and goals."

    — "Emphasis on effective, efficient, safe, and multimodal pain management plans and outcomes and a comprehensive assessment."[47] From The Official Journal of the American Society of Pain Management Nurses American Society for Pain Management Nursing and Hospice and Palliative Nurses Association, "Pain Management at the End of Life."

- I called the Hospice & Palliative Care Federation of MA, after my father died and asked them what I could have done to help my father. I was told I could have discharged him from the hospice and admitted him into a hospital.

Chapter 25
Letting Go

When they repositioned my father, his wails rode up my spine and echoed in my head like a drum beating in a canyon. The mood in my father's room grew heavier and more somber as the days passed and when nurses crossed the threshold, the tone reflected in their voices. They spoke softly and moved around quietly as my brother and I stayed anchored on each side of our father's bed.

It was Tuesday night at about 8 pm. It was dark already, and I heard Marie say hello to the nurses as she walked by them in the hallway. The lilt in her voice didn't reflect the solemn mood in the hospice. She had left Saturday morning around 10 am when Mark and I arrived. And since she was gone, my father lived in an agony that me and my brother couldn't comprehend. Her tone didn't change when she entered his room.

She asked, "How's he doing?" as she lifted her purse from across her chest.

When I turned my head to look at her, I saw she had her makeup on, and her hair was neatly pulled back and pinned in a bun. I felt my insides churning. She waltzed in like she had just arrived home after a long weekend, oblivious to the mood in the room. Marie unpacked her shopping bag of water, snacks, and her favorite magazines. And as she settled into the chair at the end of the bed, I snapped.

I said, "How do you think he's doing? He's dying."

Part of me felt bad. She had divided my family, and I hadn't gotten over it. Even with the things she had done, I wanted to believe she truly loved my father. However, my father lay dying. And she left. Not to return for three days. The nurses gave him 24 hours early Sunday morning when they called her. And despite how near he was to death, she stayed absent.

My father's room had become sacred, and in these last few hours of his life, Marie stayed with us in his room. To be in the same room with Marie meant I had to put aside her betrayals against us. We were all together for one purpose.

During the night, my father stopped breathing. First, it was brief, then the pauses stretched longer. The sounds from my father permeated the room. With each passing second, the clock on the wall seemed to tick louder, especially during the early morning hours. My father made it through another night. The following day, my brother's wife and daughter came in. They brought us some food and stayed with us for the afternoon.

My brother told his 4-year-old daughter, Grampa was sleeping while she quietly colored in her book and played with dolls in his room. It felt almost normal. When she left, with my sister-in-law, they both kissed him goodbye. And we hung up the picture she drew for him on the side of the room where I slept.

On September 11, my father's prognosis was 24 hours, again. His non-verbal pain assessment rose to ten in intensity. He couldn't verbally communicate his pain. But through his grimaced facial expressions, moaning, and clenched teeth, the nurses assessed his pain levels and intensity. The nurses observed pain both with movement and at rest. He grew guarded, and he tensed up and flinched when they moved him. It didn't matter that he begged them to stop. The nurses numbered each visit they made into his room, and they documented every single detail. On visit number twenty-six, they moved him again. And again, he cursed, swore, and screamed in pain, and he asked them to "STOP! THAT'S ENOUGH!"

My father held on for another day and on Wednesday, September 12, routine repositioning continued. Nurses followed protocol and the instructions of the hospice physician. My brother and I begged my father to please let go, and we assured him it was okay to leave.

At 10:30 pm, the nurse came. A nurse we didn't know.

I asked, "Why do you keep moving him when it causes so much pain?"

He said, "It is your choice. He doesn't have to be moved if that's what you want. It's up to you."

I said, "Why didn't somebody tell me this before?"

He said, "I don't know why."

I said, "No more moving him."

He asked me about morphine. They hadn't been giving it to him because on his chart, it stated that he was allergic. That was incorrect. Derek, the nurse, helped us to change direction. He offered solutions outside the scope of the cookie-cutter practice of moving my father every four hours. He called the doctor and called him back again until my father's pain got under control.

It was midnight and my father grew weaker. When my brother picked up his hand, my father couldn't hold on. His face had no expression. His jaw had dropped open. The intervals between breathing in and breathing out became longer. So much so that I thought he had taken his last breath more than once.

We felt like my father could go at any minute. I sat beside him, then laid down for a minute on the floor to close my eyes and stretch my back. My brother had the ball game on low volume on the TV. When I got up to use the bathroom, I walked by Marie. She was playing solitaire on her phone. I laid back down and dozed off. At 2:10 am I jumped up.

I said, "Was that it, John?"

I thought my father had taken his last breath. It wasn't what I expected. It was so soft, almost like a puff of a whisper. I ran out into the hallway.

"Derek, I think my father's gone."

He rushed in and listened to his chest. His heart was still beating.

Derek said, "We have a few minutes before his heart will stop. I'll be back in a few minutes and give you all some time to say goodbye."

I stood on the left shoulder of my father, my brother on his right. Marie came to his feet. My brother kissed his forehead and held onto his hand. My right rested on his shoulder, and Marie placed her hands on his feet. Derek stepped back into the room to check his pulse 15 minutes later. My father's heart had stopped beating. The pain was over.

I asked Derek, "What do I do next? Do I call the funeral home?"

He said, "I can do it if you like. It's up to you."

I called them. The funeral home answering service said, "The undertaker will arrive within an hour."

In the meantime, the nurses came in to prepare my father's body and asked us to step into the hallway for a few minutes. Marie went into the private room where I had met with the nurse manager and social worker. My brother and I stood around the corner near the hallway, on the edge of the waiting area. When Marie came out, I asked her if she wanted some time by herself with my father. She went in first. My brother went in next, then me. Then we came together again in his room. My brother asked Marie if she wanted to call her daughter. It was 3 am and a long ride back to the Cape. Her daughter lived halfway between where we were and the Cape. She could have stayed with them, but she wanted to drive home. Marie packed up her things.

She said, "I'll be in touch."

My brother and I said, "Goodbye. We'll talk soon."

My brother said, "Be careful driving."

Marie left our father's room.

My brother John said to me, "I'm going to wait."

I'm glad he said that because I never thought to wait. It's kind of strange in a way, but I wasn't thinking of sitting and waiting for the funeral home to arrive. I had cracked the window and the door earlier to free his soul. Then I sat with my hands on my father's feet. My brother stroked my father's head and kissed him on the forehead. The rain had eased up outside and muggy air drifted in. We sat and talked about how unreal this all seemed, and then I heard the bell ring from upstairs at the main entrance. Once, then twice, no one answered it. I knew it must have been the funeral home. I ran up the stairs to let them in and told them where my father was. They asked if I wanted to ride down in the elevator with them. Oddly, this felt comforting.

They asked us to stay outside the room while they prepared his body for transport. We heard the zipper of the bag and then the wheels of the gurney as it moved towards us in the hallway. The two men shook our hands and said they were sorry for our loss. A velvety soft blanket covered the body bag, outlining my father's frame. We couldn't resist laying our hands on him, thinking it was our last goodbye before we left. But then the undertaker asked us if we wanted to ride up in the service elevator with them. We did what most families don't do, and I'm so glad they invited us to ride along.

Before we exited the building, Derek asked our permission to perform a small spiritual ritual with the other nurse who had cared for my father. He blessed my father and honored his life with a few words. He tapped a chime, and we bowed our heads in a moment of silence. Then he brought our attention back as the low hum dissipated over my father's body. We thanked them, said goodbye, and watched as they rolled my father's body into the white hearse.

My father died on the thirteenth, the same day as my mother. It was a powerful sign. Dying was not something my father wanted, and he fought to take every breath. He left when he was ready, but even then, I don't think he was ever ready to say goodbye.

My father, John J. Sullivan Jr. died on September 13, 2018. My father hung on for days when he should have been gone. My father now shares number 13 with my mother. Their sign they use to communicate with my brother and me. They see us. They hear us. They know when we need the sign. The number 13 is a powerful connection to our parents. When we see it, we know it is them. They still guide us. And they love us as we love them. Always.

LESSONS LEARNED

- "Research from the University of New South Wales has raised questions about the correct way to care for those requiring pressure area care. The common practice of repositioning every two hours can cause patients to become more agitated and distressed." From Hellocare.'"Two-Hourly Repositioning to Prevent Bedsores Is 'Abuse.'"

- "The practice of repositioning fails to prevent bedsores from developing. The fact that the practice continues is a form of unintentional institutional elder abuse."

- "Rather than two-hourly repositioning, the researchers recommend that those assessed as being at risk of developing bedsores be given alternating-pressure air mattresses."
- "These air mattresses have been shown to prevent bedsores. This research dates back to 1967."
- "The conclusion is pressure relief should be provided in the form of an alternating-pressure air mattress."[48] From Hellocare. "Two-Hourly Repositioning to Prevent Bedsores Is 'Abuse.'"

Chapter 26

Tribute

A solid line ran through my father from the soles of his feet out through the top of his head. He aligned himself with a code of high morals, and values. He stayed true to who he was and what he believed. And the impression he left behind.... —is best described by others.

The tribute wall from the funeral home website:

> *I was truly blessed to have met Jack through Mike, George, and Joe. I have some unforgettable memories from a wonderful trip through parts of Europe and Jack opening up his house and family to us. Jack's heart was larger than life, just like his smile. Jack's firehouse stories and experiences were none less than the description of a true hero with numerous lives. Jack's expressions when eating good food and desserts always made me laugh. The best was watching Jack light up with love when he would talk about his family. You will be missed but never forgotten.*
>
> Love, Dave

My father was known as Sully in the Boston Fire Department. The following tribute is from a firefighter family.

> *We are saddened to hear of Sully's passing. My father and John were best of friends. I remember meeting him when I was a young kid and thinking*

> to myself that he was bigger than life. My brother, Jim and Sully were appointed to the B.F.D. on the same day and carpooled to the academy together. In later years, I was appointed to the B.F.D. And was fortunate enough to have worked with John a few times. Rest easy, Sully, you left a great impression behind. God bless, The Ranahan family.

From Mike, who my father met on the Big Ride Across America. They were strangers when they met and by day 48, they were family.

> To the most amazing man I have ever met. Jack, you are truly the best, tough as nails, strong as ten men, compassionate, and loving. They broke the mold with you. As you used to tell me, "The days of iron men and wooden ships are over." You were truly an "iron man." My life is better because you were my friend. Until I see you again. Love you, Mike.

From my brother's good friend.

> I was very sad to hear about Mr. Sullivan passing away. He was always smiling and laughing and had one hell of a handshake. Mr. Sullivan was a class act all the way and carried himself with great style, from the Versace ties to the always shiny Cadillac. I will always remember the fun times in his kitchen or on the couch in West Roxbury talking about and watching the Red Sox...he will be missed. My deepest sympathy to the Sullivan family. G. O. & Family

From Lauren, their friendship grew from the first year my father rode in the Pan-Mass Challenge.

> *Jack was one of the kindest, sweetest most noble men I have ever known. Every time he greeted me, he would pick me up and give me the most amazing hug! He was a top-shelf gentleman who loved life in every way. In his sad passing, I will reflect on his many virtues and kind spirit and try to bring his "Jackness" into my life. I am honored to know him. Love to his family. Lauren*

⸎

My father bought a double burial plot outside the city, in a small rural town where I used to live. My mother wanted to be buried in a place where we could always visit, away from the crime in the city, which she felt would eventually expand. Norfolk Cemetery dates back to circa 1745. A stone wall surrounds the grounds and my parents' headstone is visible from the street. The top of the square black polished granite slopes slightly, from left to right. It stands out next to the natural light grey and black and white stones near it. On the front, the name Sullivan is etched into the clouds of a blue sky with a log cabin woodland scene. A handsome buck looks out, past my mother as she leans against a large rock watching my father, brother and I fly fishing in the stream. Near her, on top of a flat boulder extending out from the shore is a raccoon standing with one leg up and claws extended. On the opposite shore, the log cabin. Downstream, a rabbit sits poised on an old fallen tree. On the back of the headstone are the lyrics from The Dance, recorded by Garth Brooks. I watched the music video of this song with my mother in 1990, two years before she died. While I watched it, I thought of all the pain she endured from cancer. I knew, then, that someday we would play this song for her. When my father was ready to pick out the stone, we inscribed the entire song on the back.

⸎

Marie knew where my father planned to be buried. And we talked about where to have the wake before he went into hospice. I wasn't sure at the time where to have it, because we lived all spread out from one another. I found a funeral home in Holden and explained to Marie where it was. She said she was fine with it. I also asked her before my father died, if she wanted to send me some pictures that she'd like to add for the wake. Marie didn't send me any. Instead, she chose to add them later to the memorial page on the funeral home's website.

My brother and I went to the funeral home the morning my father died and chose the casket. It was maple, simple, yet strong, and unassuming. The funeral home engraved a Maltese Cross, the emblem representing firefighting, into the cover, and we added Marine Corps and firefighter keepsake markers on each corner of the casket.

The funeral coordinator invited us to fill the room with personal items and pictures.

She said, "It's a big room, bring as much as you want."

Well, my brother took that and ran with it. He filled the bed of his pickup and inside the cab. He brought every piece of my father that depicted who he was and the people he loved.

The coordinator said, "Just bring them and we will set it all up for you."

My sister-in-law made collages from our family photos and photographed my father's helmet for one of his prayer cards. My brother and I had two amazing pictures. The other was a picture of my father on a bike trip. He was sitting on the side of a road with his back against a mountain range that reached the sky. We couldn't decide between the two, so we had both.

While my brother and I worked on the rest of the details for the wake, Mark called firefighter friends and asked for volunteers to stand as honor guard at the casket. Mark also found a bagpiper who volunteered for the funeral at the church.

My brother and I visited the church to go over the details of the mass. The coordinator remarked how stifling the church was this summer, causing some parishioners to feel faint. The heat didn't let up in September, so my brother and I suggested we bring coolers filled with iced water, and mints for people as they entered the church.

The coordinator spoke to my brother about his eulogy. She suggested shorter is better and she asked him to touch on my father's faith. Then she gave us a funeral worksheet to take home and fill in the names of those participating in the mass.

I texted Marie when I got home later that day. I asked if her daughter and grandsons wanted to participate in the mass, which they did.

The day of the wake my brother arrived a couple hours early. Mark and I arrived about an hour after him. We had a large group of uniformed firefighters, and so many showed up, they took shifts. Boston Fire Department sent their honor guard, and the Marines sent theirs.

When we walked into the entrance of my father's wake into the visitation room, it felt like we walked into a time capsule. The funeral coordinator had displayed every item as if it were in a museum. My father's bicycle looked ready to ride, with his helmet on the handlebars, and bike shoes next to the pedals, all set to click in. His leather suitcase lay open with his concrete trawls. Tired and well-worn concrete-dusted work boots, sat beside them, unlaced, after a hard day's work. His charred leather fire helmet was placed up on a pedestal. The brittle dried edges of the brim exposed the wire underneath. By the look of it, you knew it had seen some serious fire and been through some horrific scenes. It captured an era of courage and bravery. The continuous looping of the twenty-two-minute photo tribute captured my father's humor and vibrance. His spirit was with us.

Marie arrived with her family. She stood at the beginning of the line next to my father's casket and her grandsons took turns standing next to her. My brother and sister-in-law were next, and at the end, me and Mark. In the hallway corner behind the door to our room, my niece and her cousin played with some toys on top of a blanket.

Two firefighters from Meetinghouse Hill Firehouse sat with us and recounted the many fires, and wild, dangerous nights, they experienced as rookies. They shared what they learned working with my father. One firefighter's long-time girlfriend recounted her memories of my mother and the lasting impressions she left with her. Close friends of my brother came, and one traveled from Florida. George flew in from California. Others drove varied distances between one and four hours. Pan-Mass Challenge riders, and newer friends I had made through Mark, all paid their respects. Friends who Marie and my father grew to know over their years together paid theirs. We appreciated everyone who took time out of their lives and gave us their support with a kind word, a mass card, a note, and a hug. All helped us grieve, from the firefighters who stood at the casket, to the bagpiper, friends, and our family.

My father's love for us expanded into the room. It brought all of us together. We were forever connected because of one man.

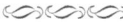

Murray, my father's friend, and partner, stayed with Mark and me at our house that night. Marie stayed with her family, not too far away. My brother and his family went home. The next morning would be our final goodbye.

Mark and I met my brother and his family at the funeral home. Many met us at the church instead of following in a procession. We stopped at Dunks for a coffee about two minutes from the church. We were the first ones to pull into the parking lot. The mass coordinator came out of the rectory to greet us when she saw us carrying the coolers. She went over the details of the mass, confirmed the names of the people who were reading the gospel, and showed us the pews for our family to sit.

The director of the funeral home got our attention next. He coordinated the procession into and out of the church like a conductor of an orchestra. He gathered the pallbearers in the back of the church and then instructed us when to go to the hearse. We had eight, my brother, my cousin Jack, Mark, George from California, Murray, Marie's two grandsons, and me.

The bagpiper played through the drizzle and fog as we carried our father's casket from the hearse and up the granite front stairs of the church. My brother stood on one front corner and me on the other. Mark was behind me and my cousin Jack, to his left, George, Murray, and Marie's grandsons were behind them. Like a blanket, we covered the sides, front, and back of our father's casket as we slowly walked him down to the front of the church.

My brother wrote and read my father's eulogy, my cousin's wife and Marie's daughter read from the gospels, and Marie's grandsons carried the gifts of bread and wine to the priest for communion.

At the end of the mass, we carried our father back to the hearse. The drizzle stopped. By the time we drove around the corner to the cemetery, the sun broke through. But we arrived to find my parents' headstone lying on its back. We had no idea what caused it. No other stone toppled over.

All who attended gathered shoulder to shoulder at the gravesite. The priest said a short prayer, followed by a military gun salute. Then Taps, the most lonesome goodbye, signaled the end of an era. Through 13 folds of the American flag, silence. At the last minute, my brother asked it be presented to me. The symbol of eternal love, God, and country lay in my lap. And another one of our greatest generations was now laid to rest.

My father wrote the following in his journal, the day before the finish line, of the Big Ride. In these words, you see the man, his spirit, and his resolve.

He wrote on July 31, 1998:

> *79.8 miles*
> *Flintstone MD to Frederick MD   Day 47*
>
> *Today we start climbing out of camp with the three hardest hills of the ride. Starting six miles into today we crossed the final two Appalachian Ridges. There were five in all. So, I said how hard can it be? It was brutal, punishing, exhausting. It was hard to catch your breath. When you climbed to the top of one and came down, you were climbing another for eighty miles. This went on. I think it was on this stretch I lost most of my weight. I was soaked with sweat. All day it was pouring off me and Mike,*

but we could smell the finish line in Washington DC. Only one day to go. We are pumped up. We just want to finish. We lost so many with injuries. We were praying.

In the end, how you live your life is what you take with you to the grave. It's what you leave behind for others to remember you by. It is your character that lives on. That is your legacy.

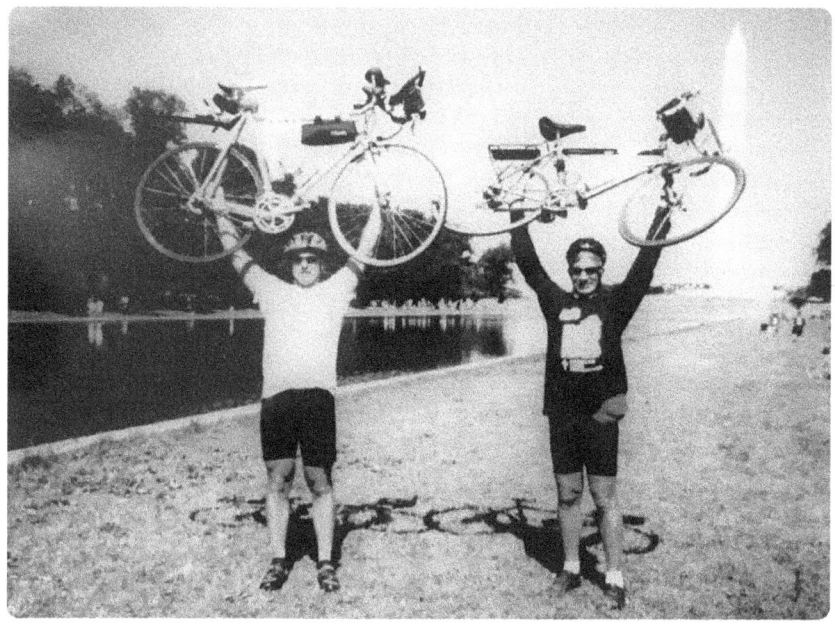

Mike Keefe and John (Jack) Sullivan taken July 31,1998, Day 48 of the Big Ride, in Washington DC. The finish. *Photo from the Sullivan Family photo collection*

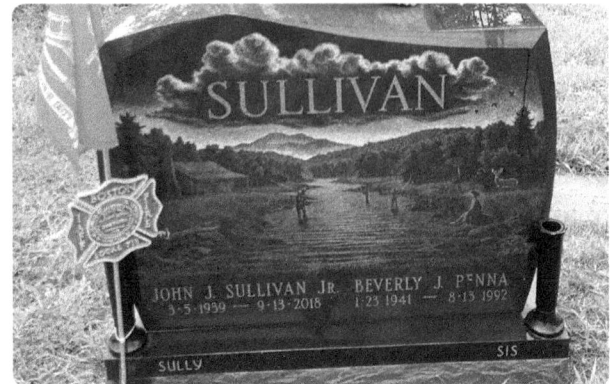

Headstone for John and Beverly (Sis) Penna Sullivan. *Photo by John Sullivan*

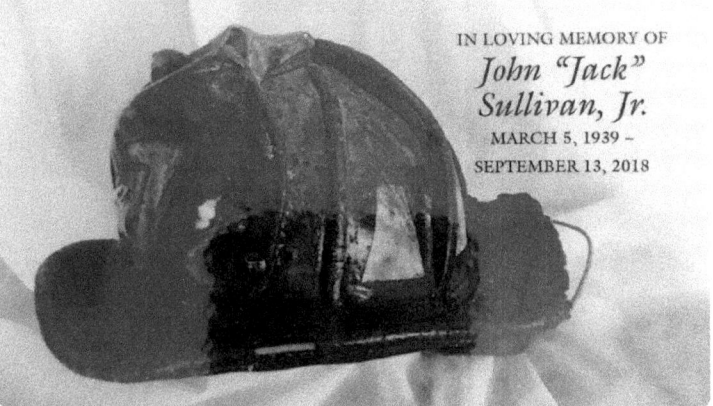

Fire Helmet - John's Prayer Card. *Photo by Karen Carone Sullivan*

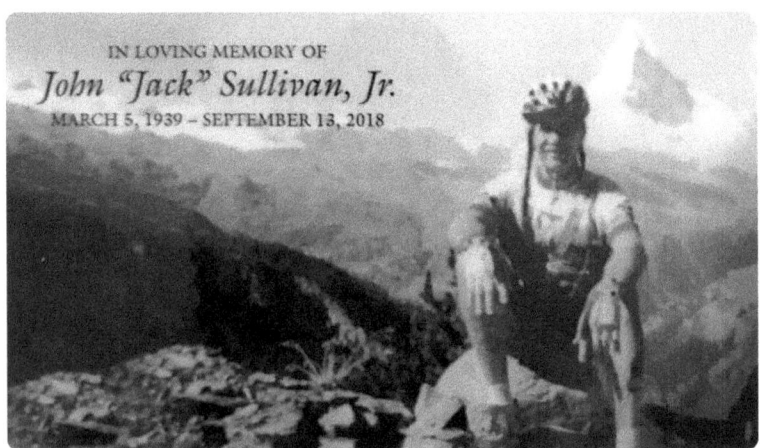

John's 2nd Prayer Card. Picture taken in Europe on a cycling trip. John was taking a break on top of a mountain in the 1990s. *From the Sullivan Family Collection*

Chapter 27

Life After

After my father's death, I hit the proverbial bottom. My body ached with sadness. And anger refused to leave my side. I couldn't close my eyes without seeing and hearing my father before his death. These visions and sounds consumed my everyday life. They made me irritable and on edge. I couldn't think of anything else. I tried to force normalcy and jump over the grieving process, and I returned to work soon after the funeral. As a massage therapist, a large part of my practice included providing healing therapies for people with cancer for a non-profit organization. My clients ranged from just-diagnosed individuals to hospice patients. When I massaged people, especially those with the same cancer as my father, I crumbled inside.

My brain couldn't make sense of the horrific pain my father endured in the hospice because it made no sense. My father went to die in a hospice home where their primary responsibility was to provide pain relief and comfort at the end of his life. However, they failed to provide what they promised. The experience was beyond comprehension.

I wanted to bury the pain of what happened to my father with him, but I couldn't. I tried, but my mind did not rest. When I drifted off to sleep, my mind went haywire. My thoughts and dreams in my sleep had merged with the same thoughts and visions when I was awake. My mind had taken on one rhythm. The recurring nightmares of not being able to help my father weren't dreams. They were a vivid representation of my reality. The last week of my father's life suffering in the hospice had embedded itself into my psyche.

So, I tried to find out more. I wanted to know how and why it happened and what I might have done differently to change the outcome. I felt compelled to make my case about my father's care. Two months after my father died, on November 19, 2018, I wrote a letter to the executive director and CEO of the hospice, and I described in horrific detail the events that took place in their hospice home from September 6 through September 13. About two weeks later, I received a call from the executive director's secretary. The executive director and she both offered their condolences. They expressed how sorry they were. The director also added that what happened to my father shouldn't have happened. She asked if I was interested in an in-person meeting with my father's physician for closure. I took some time to think about it.

I accepted her offer about three weeks later. They didn't schedule our appointment until February. I called and asked for a copy of my father's medical records from the hospice house, to prepare for my meeting. I reviewed, highlighted, and made notes on every visit. At 2, or 3, in the morning, I found myself online looking up hospital beds, hospice failures, and federal government hospice requirements. I didn't want this meeting to go to waste. I needed to know what I was talking about, and I needed to present the facts.

On December 28, 2018, I filed a consumer complaint form with the Mass. Attorney General. Their office is an advocate and resource to protect the people. On January 28, 2019, after not being able to sleep and still searching for answers, I found myself around 2 am googling the hospice physician looking for any insight into what had happened. Then I found something. Under the physician profile for the hospice physician, Dr. Barn,(not his real name), it stated in 2006 there was a voluntary agreement not to practice medicine. (non-disciplinary). On Oct.4, 2006, it stated there was a stay of suspension and probation for him. On April 20, 2011, the physician's probation was terminated, with no explanation as to why.

At 9 am the next morning, I called the Board of Registration in Medicine to request a full report. A couple of days later I received the Statement of Allegations, from the Board of Registration in Medicine, Docket No. 06-157. "The Board has reason to believe that the physician,

Dr. Barn, has committed misconduct in the practice of medicine and has violated Mass. Gen. Laws Chapter 94C and Board regulations by obtaining a controlled substance for self-use."

From the Factual Allegations, "Dr. Barn has a history of substance abuse and depression which were in remission for three years. In 2005, he experienced health problems that required surgery and the use of controlled substances to treat his post-operative pain. Shortly thereafter, he also suffered exasperation of his depression."

The record said, "Early February 2006, Dr. Barn took two prescription blanks from his colleague's prescription pad. When he took the slips, he wrote his colleague's Drug Enforcement Administration controlled substance registration number (DEA number) on one of the slips. On February 10, 2006, he prescribed himself for 15 oxycodone tablets. He filled out the prescription and used the pills."

The record continued, "On February 17, 2006, Dr. Barn wrote another oxycodone prescription for himself on the second slip he had taken from his colleague and attempted to fill it. The pharmacist questioned the prescription because it was missing the DEA number. The pharmacist notified the colleague of Dr. Barn, whose name was written on the script. The colleague reported the incident to Dr. Barn's employer. Dr. Barn took an immediate leave of absence from work and initiated treatment to recover from his relapse."

According to The Board of Registration in Medicine records, Dr. Barn's license to practice medicine was indefinitely suspended. Although, he could petition based on documentation of six months of continuous sobriety and no use of controlled substances, other than those prescribed for legitimate medical purposes along with other detailed orders as requirements.

Dr. Barn broke an ethical boundary to relieve his pain. He took an extreme measure. Dr. Barn didn't act with the same urgency to relieve my father's pain. He showed no feeling, no immediate concern, just apathy. Why did the hospice executive director allow this doctor with his background to practice with such a vulnerable population? I wanted to know.

The night before I met with the executive director of the hospice, I made a folder. In it I put an outline, copies of my father's medical chart, and, lastly, the Board of Registration in Medicine files on Dr. Barn. I had knots in my stomach. I needed to be clear and concise. But more importantly, I needed to avoid a tailspin into an emotional rant. I had to stay on point.

I was sitting in the lobby of the hospice administrative building waiting to be called for my meeting when the executive director walked by me. When the receptionist at the desk pointed me out to the executive director, she came over and introduced herself.

She said, "Hi, I'm the executive director. To my knowledge, we weren't meeting in person. I thought this was a conference call."

I said, "I understood this meeting with you and Dr. Barn was here, in person, in your office."

The receptionist at the front desk overheard me.

She said, "Dr. Barn just passed me on the stairway. I'll call him on his phone and see if I can catch him before he leaves."

I heard his phone ringing as the receptionist escorted me up to the executive director's office for our meeting. Dr. Barn didn't answer.

I stepped off the elevator on the top floor. I was told to wait in the large boardroom. The executive director's office suite was one door away. She came in and moved me to her office. She took her seat in an oversized leather chair behind a mahogany desk that took up a large corner of the room. The windows looked over a portion of the city. They scaled from floor to ceiling. It felt so removed from the hospice home. I don't know why, but the surroundings made me more nervous than I already was.

A newly hired nurse manager introduced himself. He explained he had joined the meeting, and he offered me the seat next to him. First, the executive director expressed her condolences and when she finished, I took off. I went over the details from the beginning. I read the notes from my father's chart. On the third day, meds had *some effect*. On the fourth day, *meds no longer working*, and *significant pain burden*. Pain medication was documented as *not adequate*.

I said, "My father was tough as nails, but this was torturous."

Then I explained about the employee who told my brother and me it was unethical to give too much pain medication at first.

I said, "With such ease, so matter of fact, she looked at me and said, *I know it's hard, but pain medication has to be given in increments.* She made excruciating pain sound normal. A transition that had to be endured."

I looked at the director and nurse manager for answers. They shook their heads in disbelief. I continued.

I said, "Repositioning my father inflicted pain. HE SHOUTED, SCREAMED, SWORE, and BEGGED THEM TO STOP, THAT'S ENOUGH, STOP."

I didn't realize it in the meeting then, but the nurses had typed these words in bold print on my father's medical records. I think they were trying to get the attention of the doctor.

I asked, "Was the doctor even looking at my father's chart?"

By now, Dr. Barn didn't show up at the meeting.

I said, "Dr. Barn documented in my father's medical report that he provided sixty minutes of family counseling regarding illness progression and symptom management. Dr. Barn entered the room at 11:16 am and left at 11:22 am. He asked me where I was from and if I had any brothers or sisters, and then he told me he was assessing my father. He was in and out in six minutes, not sixty like he billed Medicare for."

There was nothing the executive director could say because she honestly didn't know what to say.

I had done some research on repositioning patients and beds.

I asked, "Why couldn't they have used cushions and air mattresses, so my father didn't have to be moved?"

The new manager said, "They have those."

So, I asked again, "Why didn't they use them?"

They didn't have an answer. They didn't know why.

The director and the nurse manager said, "You could have asked for a new bed."

I said, "We did ask. We were told they didn't have one."

The director said, "They could have called out for one."

I thought to myself, *how would I have known that*?

I asked, "How old are the beds?"

The director said, "They are original to the building."

I said, "So, they are twenty years old?"

She said, "Yes."

These were heavy metal beds with steel and wire coils. They didn't tailor medical care to each person, as stated on their website. They used no alternative measures to prevent bedsores. They inflicted pain. She expressed how sorry she was again.

I asked, "Do you ever visit the hospice home?"

She replied, "No, I'm very busy."

I said, "All you have to do is grab a coffee at the hospice home on your way into your office. Being seen and present makes you approachable and gives you insight you can't get from behind a desk." Because it was evident to me through one nurse in particular, that many had the inside track on Dr. Barn. The executive director could have seen and heard for herself if she took some time to be present. But the executive director responded she was very busy and had no time to visit the hospice house. Dr. Barn never called into the meeting or showed up.

At the end of the meeting, I presented the executive director with Dr. Barn's public record from the Commonwealth of Massachusetts. By the shocked look on her face, I saw she was not aware of his history.

She asked, "May I make a copy?"

I handed it over to her.

I said, "I realize people make mistakes, but I would have thought that Dr. Barn's experience with post-operative pain and the extreme measures he went to, would have given him more compassion and an understanding of what it was like for those who are dying. No patient entering hospice, or their family, is thinking they must research the physicians who are on staff. Our minds are full, our hearts are breaking, and we trust the hospice we choose is going to fulfill the promises they made to us."

She said, "Changes are being made, and we don't usually conduct business like this."

The executive director said again, "I am very sorry."

Then the newly hired manager in the meeting asked, "Can we do anything for you?"

My voice cracked.

I said, "My father would not want anyone else to suffer the way he did. And this can't happen to someone else."

They asked me if I wanted to go to a bereavement group. A bereavement group might not touch even the surface of what I and my family had experienced. I declined and thanked them for their time.

Author's Note: The facts of the case stated here are true and can be confirmed in the Commonwealth of Massachusetts, Board of Registration in Medicine. Docket No. 06-157, Adjudicatory Case No. 2006-048. https://www.mass.gov/orgs/board-of-registration-in-medicine. To request detailed information that is not on the physician profile, borim.info@state.ma.us.

LESSONS LEARNED

I believe an executive director who rarely, if ever, steps into the hospice facility is missing a major opportunity to increase the quality of care provided.

Why? Because it's difficult for a manager to get an actual sense of what is happening inside a facility when managing from the outside. An executive director who is present at the facility gives patients, visitors, and staff a person they can reach out to when managers are not available and/or unequipped to resolve problems and handle crises, as in my father's case.

- Having a report from a manager is not the same as being there. When an executive director and/or owner visits their facility, it shows a level of care that exceeds what is written on their website or in the marketing pamphlet. It shows they have a vested interest in the quality of care that is provided and the staff who work for them.

- Staff members perform better when the management values and appreciates what they do. When staff don't feel supported, how they view and do their job can be affected.

Chapter 28
Empty Promises

I believe many complaints about hospice failure to provide pain control don't get reported to regulators. After a traumatic death, loved ones are exhausted, mentally, and physically drained. We need to mourn, be with our families, and put back our lives. I never imagined that the hospice could not provide comfort and pain control at the end of my father's life. If I had known this, I'd have discussed it with the hospice and sought an additional backup plan from the very beginning.

To file a complaint means reliving every detail. I know because I have filed them. I exhausted every resource, I spoke with, wrote to, and met with, every person who had the power to act and the voice to speak on what happened to my father. I found if the trauma doesn't break you, the bureaucracy of the system will. They handled my complaints more like a game of "kick the can down the road" than a service put in place to serve and protect the public.

It may sound like I went to extremes to seek answers and accountability. However, I wanted someone to take the initiative with a plan that involved a course correction and a commitment to ensure pain control at the end of life. That never happened through the people and organizations I contacted.

Although the hospice executive director told me changes were being made, I wanted assurance. I needed to follow through. I emailed my US Representative Jim McGovern and set up a meeting in his Worcester government office, only a couple of blocks away from the hospice headquarters.

My husband, a fire captain in the city, met me at the representative's office for the meeting. He came by to support me; he'd been on duty that day. There were four of us at the meeting: the representative, his secretary Mary Pat, myself, and my husband.

I said to the representative, "My father was a Boston firefighter. He served in the Marines. He served his community, and his country and he deserved to die in comfort as the hospice promised. The executive director said, 'It shouldn't have happened.' I would like to know if the changes she spoke of are being made. If this happened to my father, it could happen to anyone."

The representative listened, and then he told me about his experience in his own family with Alzheimer's.

He said, "It's awful. It's sad. What I can do is meet with the executive director. Then I will contact you afterward and the three of us will follow up with a final meeting."

I said, "That would be great. Thank you. I appreciate it. I look forward to meeting again."

I thought I had made progress, and I had a good feeling about our upcoming meeting. Five weeks went by. I hadn't heard from Representative McGovern or his office secretary who had given me her card. When I didn't hear from either of them, I reached out. I called, emailed, and left a voicemail and explained my follow-up. Then four months went by. Still no reply. I believed him. I felt that he genuinely cared, and I didn't want to give up on him.

The only other person I could think of who might speak to him on my behalf was the Worcester City Manager. I emailed his office and explained what occurred in the hospice house and my meeting with Representative McGovern.

The city manager said, "I believe you've checked all the right boxes and spoken to the right people. I'm sorry you're not getting the action and attention merited by this situation."

Representative McGovern, and his secretary, never returned my calls or emails. I had to accept their silence as their response. It was my cue to move on.

I searched online for organizations and people involved with the rights and safety of people living with Alzheimer's. I found the Bipartisan

Congressional Task Force for Alzheimer's. It's an organization that is involved in legislation and raising public awareness. Their other priorities include changing the way the nation addresses Alzheimer's.

I sent a letter to three US senators listed on the Task Force for Alzheimer's website, https://alzimpact.org/task_force:, Senator Edward Markey, Senator Susan Collins, and Senator Joe Kennedy.

I addressed the physical pain my father experienced in the hospice home. I stated that end-of-life care needs to be addressed with an alternative plan of care for loved ones and families where hospice cannot provide pain relief. I also touched on the security and protection needs of people living with Alzheimer's and the solutions I had that could be expanded upon. However, Senator Markey, Senator Collins, and Senator Joe Kennedy have yet to respond.

Then I filed a consumer complaint with the Massachusetts Attorney General on December 28, 2018, on the hospice house and Dr. Barn. After six weeks, the attorney general's office sent me a letter informing me that they decided my complaint should be handled by a different department. They shuffled it down to the Health and Human Services Department and thanked me for bringing my concerns to their attention. The attorney general closed my complaint without ever opening it. For months my complaint seemed to be held in suspended animation. I followed up with the Massachusetts Department of Public Health on July 10, 2019. The person who answered the call didn't identify who they were or their department.

I asked, "Is this The Division of Health Care Facility Licensure and Certification of the Department of Public Health?"

The man said, "Ya."

I said, "The attorney general's office sent my complaint here on February 11."

Then I explained my complaint.

The man, said, "Ya, we don't do that here."

I asked, "Do I have the right number? 800-462-5540?"

The man said, "You have the right number, but I can't help you."

I hung up and almost gave up. But I thought, maybe the governor's office? Maybe, they will listen or take some action.

I sent a letter to Governor Charles D. Baker's office explaining the failures in the medical system and the details of what occurred to my father. Their office replied. *Thank you for your input.* Next, I emailed and called attorneys and asked if what happened to my father in the hospice fell under malpractice and negligence.

I said, "Dr. Barn should not have been working in the hospice. He failed to provide pain management and under his direction pain was inflicted over and over again through repositioning."

However, medical malpractice attorneys did not consider it a case of malpractice. My father's death was not directly caused by the intense pain they inflicted. Neither the physician nor the hospice was liable. They did not cause his death. Therefore, it was not malpractice.

I hung up the phone and my mind and my body ceased. As my breath left my chest, the memories of my father's pain surged through me like a fast-moving stream in a spring flood. I sat paralyzed, staring out the window. Then pools of water rushed down my cheeks. And in the stillness, my mind filled with the visions of my father squeezing the rail of the hospice bed with all his might.

Months went by and I kept wondering if I had missed something and if there was anyone else, I could have contacted. Then on July 9, 2019, I heard a news report that revealed the results of a four-year investigation into hospices across the country.

"The reports are the government's first to look at hospice deficiencies nationwide. The Office of the Inspector General in the Department of Health and Human Services found that from 2012 through 2016, health inspectors cited 87% of hospices for deficiencies. And 20% of hospices had lapses serious enough to endanger patients."[49] From the Office of The Inspector General, "Vulnerabilities in the Medicare Hospice Program Affect Quality Care and Program Integrity: An OIG Portfolio." 2018b. Office of Inspector General | Government Oversight | US Department of Health and Human Services.

"The Office of the Inspector General found that hospices do not always provide needed services to beneficiaries and sometimes provide poor quality care. In some cases, hospices were not able to manage effectively symptoms or medications, leaving beneficiaries in unnecessary pain for many days."[50] From the Office of The Inspector General, "Vulnerabilities in the Medicare Hospice Program Affect

Quality Care and Program Integrity: An OIG Portfolio." 2018b. Office of Inspector General | Government Oversight | US Department of Health and Human Services.

Now there was evidence. What happened to my father wasn't an isolated event. There were others whose loved ones had suffered due to a lack of pain control by hospices. Since it was in the news, I thought for sure what happened to him would now emit a response other than, *case closed.*

I emailed the Inspector General in Washington, DC on Friday, July 19, 2019, and described in detail the events at the hospice house. In my email, I told her that the pain my father endured while under hospice care was unconscionable. I went through each person I contacted up to this point, including my meeting with Jim McGovern, my Massachusetts member of Congress. I told her I felt as though the system was broken, and I quoted the Federal Register which stated "Circumstances during the end-of-life may necessitate short-term inpatient admission to a hospital, skilled nursing facility, or hospice facility for procedures necessary for pain control or acute or chronic symptom management that cannot be managed in any other setting. These acute hospice care services are to *ensure* that any new or worsening symptoms are intensively addressed."[51] From the "Medicare Program; FY 2018 Hospice Wage Index and Payment Rate Update and Hospice Quality Reporting Requirements."

I said in my email, "I felt as though my complaint has been pushed aside and sent down the proverbial bureaucratic political chain and held in a perpetual state of gridlock. (No offense to you.)"

On September 12, 2019, two months after I submitted my complaint, the Office of the Inspector General responded I should contact the Centers for Medicare & Medicaid Services (CMS), New York Regional Office, Division of Survey and Certification (DSC). They also forwarded my complaint to the Acting Associate Regional Administrator for the New York DSC for review and provided me with follow-up contact information.

Dr. Barn took his 6 minutes of counseling and billed Medicare 60. Asking me where my father was from is not counseling and neither was asking me if I had any brothers or sisters. Dr. Barn seemed to prioritize remitting his billable hours over pain relief. I wasn't concerned about counseling. I wanted Dr. Barn to care about relieving my father from his pain. I wanted him to voluntarily stand up and take responsibility for not fulfilling his obligations as a hospice physician.

The Office of the Inspector General referred this matter to the Centers for Medicare and Medicaid Services Boston Regional Office, Division of Financial Management and Fee for Service Operations. My complaint was forwarded by the Office of the Inspector General to an Associate Regional Administrator, and they provided me with follow-up contacts. They conveyed their deep commitment, and the Office of the Inspector General assured me of the integrity and effectiveness of all the programs of HHS. They also thanked me for bringing this matter to their attention. After reviewing my case, the result was that there were no violations or deficiencies found. Dr. Barn billed Medicare for 60 minutes for zero counseling. Again, this revealed how the system leaned in to protect the physician.

Every person and organization I contacted had a responsibility to protect and advocate for the rights of the people, to determine what is just, and to call out what is wrongful. At the bare minimum, I thought they would at least attempt to. However, in their eyes, they believed they had done their job.

> On Jul 19, 2019, at 3:54 PM, City Manager < wrote:
>
> Good afternoon Ms. Wyco,
>
> Thank you for contacting the Office of the City Manager. I want to start by expressing my condolences for your loss. Saying that the actions of ▓▓▓ Hospice House's employees made a terrible situation worse is an understatement. After reading your letter, it sounds like you're an excellent advocate for any coming behind you, as you work to ensure these mistakes won't happen again. I believe you've checked all the right boxes and spoke to the right people. I'm sorry you're not getting the action and attention merited by this situation. What can the City do to assist you? I don't believe we license hospice care facilities; they may be licensed with the State. Similarly, the City doesn't do much against medical professionals that shouldn't be practicing; something like that is way out of our jurisdiction.
>
> If you think I can help answer questions or connect you with another agency or service provider, please do not hesitate to reach out at any time. Please take care.
>
> Joshua Martunas
> Staff Assistant & Records Access Officer
> Office of the City Manager Edward M. Augustus, Jr.
> P: 508-799-1175 ext. 31302
> F: 508-799-1208

July 19, 2019 Email to Jacqueline from the Office of the City Manager. *From the author's records.*

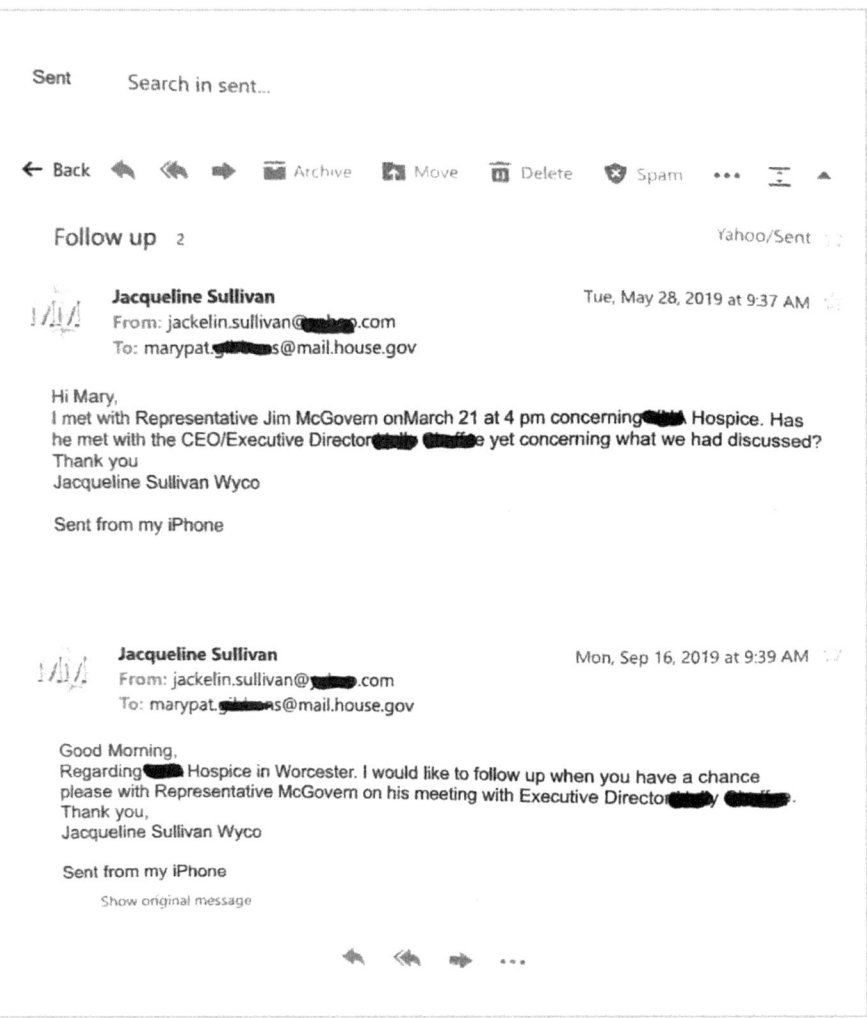

May 28, 2019 and Sept 16, 2019 emails from Jacqueline to Representative McGovern's Secretary, Mary Pat. *From the author's records.*

Chapter 29
Healing

I was hellbent on seeking answers since my father died on September 13, 2018. But one day shy of the first anniversary of this death, I gave up and ended my pursuit of accountability of the hospice facility and the hospice physician. Every attorney I spoke with said *there is no case*.

My father's hospice physician, along with the executive director of the hospice, escaped accountability as my father's death was not a direct consequence of their actions. In the eyes of the law, they were untouchable. And is was unanimous. Attorneys never said the words, but the implied that I accept it and move on.

Do No Harm, the core principle of the Hippocratic Oath, protected Dr. Barn, not my father. In my mind, it wasn't morally or ethically right. I didn't know how I was supposed to take this and live with it and my grief came to an abrupt halt. The anger blocked everything else out in my life. On September 12, 2019, I arrived exactly were I started. I had no one left to call and nowhere else to turn, and that's when I began to write this book.

As for Marie, my relationship with her ended in March 2018, six months before my father died, when she dared me to bring my father home. I said goodbye to Marie at the luncheon after my father's funeral. It was the last time I saw her. An attorney speaks for me when needed.

My brother John and sister-in-law Karen have two children. Their daughter and son are my parents' namesakes. Jack was born about a year after my father died. My husband Mark was on duty at a three-alarm fire on November 13, 2019, when two firefighters got trapped. Mark narrowly made it out, and one firefighter died. The effects of the cumulative tragedies throughout his career led to post-traumatic stress and prevented him from returning to the job. He retired.

The healing is ongoing. I don't think it will ever be completed. Writing this book has given me as much comfort as it has deep sadness and outrage. Advocates who are currently speaking for people with Alzheimer's can't wait for the legal system to catch up to protect their loved ones. I believe when you learn how to detect emotional harm and financial exploitation, you will be able to stop it and prevent it.

In life, my father guided me. And after his death, he entered my innermost thoughts. He makes his presence known in multiple ways. There are days when the same white car he drove goes past me as I think of him. Yes, it could be just a coincidence, but instantly another sign appears like a Boston firefighter sticker on a car or a bike rider wearing a shirt with Boston or the Pan-Mass Challenge. There are days I smile because the connection is astonishing. A truck with the name Sullivan lettered on the side drives by, and then Keystone, the street where I grew up, appears on a sign. A lady walks past me and says *Dad*, as she is talking on the phone. The TV is on in the background, while I'm reliving the worst days of my father's life. The actors on the screen reminisce about their father, *he was one of a kind, so strong. His family meant everything to him.* My father doubles and triples his signs to communicate with me, so there is no mistaking that I know it is him. The number 13 ebbs and flows throughout my days. Whether it's on a license plate in front of me as I'm driving, or on my receipts from the store, it's a constant and ever-present sign of our connection.

I felt my father's presence on the day I had to accept that no one would help me find the answers or assume accountability. My father's identity was replaced with a number on a docket. The agony he endured in hospice that was preventable went into a case file. And who he was became irrelevant.

I wanted those I contacted and others I filed complaints with to imagine if they were going through what my father had. I wrote the following poem. I believe every word came from my father. I used pieces of it throughout my book because I wasn't sure to include it. It seemed too sad. But I feel you have a great sense of who my father was, and you will understand the meaning behind these words.

Reeling Inside and Coming to Terms

What if it were you?
Don't snicker at the man who forgets his name
 or where he lives,
Or stumbles to find the right words to say.
Unless you live in the mind that betrays him every day.
When he is lost where he once knew
Don't scorn him and insist that he knows.
For he does not, anymore
What if it were you? How would you feel?
Would you feel shame? Would it cause you to hide
 your head?
What if it were you?
Would you fear the same fate?
Could you withstand the awkward stares?
And the whispers of others as you walk in the room?
They have no idea the hell you are in
For a smile is worn for all to see while tears weep
 silently inside
The future does not exist, not anymore.
Once I saw my children and my children's children,
And theirs
Once there were plans
Where shall we go? What shall we see?
When we retire, there it will all be just waiting for us to see.
Not any more
Now I see nothing.
Only the end,
The end, I thought that was so far away.
Is nearer than I could have imagined.
What will happen to me?
Will I be put away?
Locked in a room.
Unable to go where I once went.
What will happen to me?

Fear Knocked — Jacqueline Sullivan Wyco

Will I be alone for days on end?
Not knowing where I am
Will anyone care?
How will my life end?
My life was full of promise.
Alzheimer's stole it from me.
I don't ask "Why me?"
I ask only why this disease exists.
How cruel?
No one escapes.
Life without challenge
This is the hand I was dealt.
So, I must face my fate.
I have to prepare.
Take care of my family.
For it is them, I'm most proud.
I wish for them everything in life because they are
    my greatest achievement.
I have made my decisions and put into place those who
    will carry out my mission.
To them, I trust wholeheartedly.
They will abide by me, I know.
Let them be strong and happy and live a life well lived,
    for it is I who have done just that.
I pray no force will stand in the way of
    my long-term decisions.
For if it does
I pray for the strength of my advocates
    to carry them through.
I fear pain, let me die in peace.
With my family by my side,

I don't want to go, and my urge to fight to live is strong.
Giving up is not something I know how to do.
It's not how I'm made.
But I know it is something I must do,
I'll fight to take every breath.
You can count on that.
I'll fight to the end.
I'll leave when I'm ready. Not a moment before
And even then
I don't think I will be.
Ever ready to say goodbye.
When my body fails, I'll have no choice.
And when I am gone
I'll see everything.
The past will be clear.
I'll be whole again.
And there I'll be.
With you
My family, my children, and my children's children
I'll be here with you.
Always near
Have no fear.
Now, close your eyes. And imagine. What if it were you?

—Author—Jacqueline Sullivan Wyco

Chapter 30
Advocates and Advanced Directives

An Alzheimer's diagnosis doesn't come with an instruction manual. There aren't seminars, workshops, or continuing education classes along the stages of the disease to help advocates, family members, and those who are diagnosed with Alzheimer's. And maybe there should be.

A person who is diagnosed with Alzheimer's will need to prepare advanced directives and name their advocates. A good solid advocate is crucial to advanced directives for long-term protection and security.

However, choosing a loved one, or family member, as an advocate requires some forethought. A person's traits and behavioral patterns can predict how they may act as an advocate.

In my opinion, there are personality traits to consider when selecting advocates. An advocate:

- is a person who has integrity. They are truthful and take responsibility for their actions.
- is loyal.
- is reliable.
- remains compassionate and calm under stress.
- respects rights and boundaries of others.
- follows directions.

I believe an advocate needs to be balanced with their ability to empathize, listen, and communicate without judgment. This is not always easy, especially when family members or professionals try to persuade advocates to modify or alter decisions made by the person with Alzheimer's. An Alzheimer's advocate is a person who believes that the decisions of the person with Alzheimer's takes precedence over what others think or feel. Ultimately, an advocate must be engrained with an uncompromising ability to stand up for and carry out the person's decisions regardless of the beliefs and views of others.

Protection and security of the person with Alzheimer's is paramount. I firmly believe that if we are to deter and stop abuse, we must think of choosing an advocate like filling a position for a job.

There are specific personality traits that don't make the best choice for an advocate. I was unaware that there are clusters of characteristics associated with a personality type that could predict abuse. This led me to analyze traits and behavioral patterns.

"Narcissism is the personality type most prone to secret abuse," says Psychology Today. In the last few decades, researchers have been measuring a cluster of traits ready-made to predict abuse — the Dark Tetrad, a frankly exploitative, aggressive type marked by four traits:

1. narcissism, best thought of as the drive to feel special.

2. psychopathy, a pattern of remorseless lies and manipulation.

3. Machiavellianism, a cold, chess-playing approach to life and love.

4. sadism, a troubling tendency to delight in the suffering of others.

Some of these traits are patently more dangerous than others. In decades of studies on bullying and aggression, one aspect of pathological narcissism — exploitation and entitlement — predicts just about every nasty behavior documented, including physical abuse, and chronic lies."[52] From Psychology Today, "What Everyone Should Know about Covert Abusers."
"Recognizing covert narcissism requires looking beyond obvious appearances, past common assumptions and expectations. For this reason, covert narcissism is more difficult to spot, and it can take years to recognize it in someone you think you know well. The more covert form of pathological narcissism and narcissistic personality disorder is not expressed the same way in every individual, but there

are typical patterns that are very common. If you see many or most of these attitudes and behaviors in a person you know, you're probably dealing with someone who suffers—and makes others suffer—with covert narcissism.

1. Is passive-aggressive
2. Criticizes and judges from the sidelines
3. Is condescending and superior
4. Is threatened by honesty and directness
5. Swings between idealizing and devaluing him-/herself and others
6. Denies and dismisses others' feelings
7. Cultivates a public image sharply different from his/her private behavior
8. Identifies as a victim
9. Is cynical and sarcastic
10. Makes unreasonable demands
11. Turns your problems into his/her dramas
12. Belittles and blames
13. Exploits and/or attacks others' vulnerability
14. Is reactive to questioning or criticism
15. Plays on sympathies
16. Fakes or exaggerates illness/injury for attention
17. Withholds and stonewalls
18. Gaslights
19. Avoids introspection and lacks self-awareness
20. Uses platitudes in place of genuine insight
21. Denies own anger
22. Focuses on unfairness
23. Is envious and vengeful
24. Prefers to remain behind the scenes
25. Gossips
26. Triangulates
27. Holds a grudge
28. Needs reassurance
29. Is inattentive or annoyed when others talk

30. Has double standards
31. Hates to lose
32. Fixates on others' problems and misfortunes
33. Flatters and fawns to win favor
34. Displays rage and contempt in private
35. Resists decision-making
36. Does not sincerely apologize
37. Avoids direct responsibility, shifts blame onto others
38. Has an exaggerated sense of entitlement
39. Is impressed by the overt narcissist's appearance of confidence
40. Lacks emotional empathy
41. Focuses on appearance over substance
42. Rushes to (false) intimacy
43. Is anxious and hypervigilant
44. Displays false humility and humblebrags
45. Is prone to paranoia and conspiracy theories
46. Crosses normative boundaries and codes of conduct
47. Pokes, prods, and pries
48. Feels special through association
49. Feels above the rules
50. Uses guilt, silent treatment, and shame to control and punish
51. Expects caretaking
52. Conducts smear campaigns"[53]

From Psychology Today, "52 Ways to Identify a Covert Narcissist."

Most will agree that these traits and behavioral patterns would be problematic in an advocate. Be objective if considering the older child, sibling, spouse, or other loved family member as an advocate. Is their temperament, personality, and character the best fit for the job?

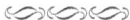

Advanced Directives

The decisions of healthcare proxies and living wills for people with Alzheimer's are at risk of becoming null and void. An advocate who is doing their due diligence, and the directives themselves, are not enough protection.

My father chose his advocate and decided the terms and conditions of his future healthcare decisions. It was his right. However, his primary care physician overrode his decision to have me speak for him as his advocate. She refused to communicate with me about ongoing medical treatments for him. I filed a formal complaint with the Massachusetts Board of Registration in Medicine. The result: she was not liable for not adhering to my father's healthcare proxy. Her opinions, morals, and beliefs overrode those of my father's. In her reply to my complaint she said, "Whether or not a patient's proxy is in place, I will involve family, to complete medical forms, regardless of a patient's legal right to have their medical choices voiced and upheld by their chosen advocate."

Healthcare advocates of people with Alzheimer's must know that healthcare directives are not binding. The Massachusetts Board of Registration in Medicine determined my complaint, docket #18-312, against my father's primary care physician, warranted no disciplinary action. My father's legal right to have me speak for him and make decisions based on his values and beliefs was overridden and disregarded. His case was closed.

Here are some things to consider, according to Compassion and Choices, Advanced Care Planning.

What are the Limitations of Advance Directives?

- "Lack of enforcement: Most states grant doctors legal protection. Physicians have little incentive to follow advanced directives. They are more likely to revert to training and do everything possible to keep a terminally ill person alive, regardless of whether the treatment only prolongs an agonizing dying process." I suggest, if the person's current physician and/or facility cannot honor the person's end-of-life decisions, reach out to your social worker. They have the networking capability and resources to help you find a physician and facility that will.

- "Lack of Access: If advanced directives are locked away and when an emergency happens family members and physicians may be unaware, that they exist."
- "Lack of relevance: When documents are made years in advance, they can lack relevance to current events and circumstances."
- "Lack of dialogue: Instructions on paper are mostly ineffective unless the people authorized to give them the effect know in advance what the instructions say."[54] From Compassion and Choices, "Advance Care Planning." This is why advocates need to record, document, and communicate from the onset of Alzheimer's diagnosis and along every stage of the disease. In addition, there are forms including a Dementia addendum to improve the chances that advanced directives will be honored on the Compassion and Choices webpage, https://compassionandchoices.org/our-issues/advance-care-planning/.
- Consider the fact that people afflicted with Alzheimer's can live for many years. I suggest advanced directives state where the person wants to reside. And at what stage of the disease.
- Look at the person's health history and family history. Consider if the person with Alzheimer's is diagnosed with another terminal illness such as lung, pancreatic, or breast cancer: The stage of cancer, life expectancy, and prognosis are part of the decision-making process. Be specific in directives. At what stage does the person wish to receive or decline treatment?

- What about chronic conditions such as kidney disease? Does the person wish to receive dialysis?
- What about consent for surgeries such as heart, intestinal blockages, aneurysms, and blood clots?

Having an advanced directive does not guarantee that end-of-life instructions will be honored. But advocates can significantly increase the odds by:

- being present at all appointments.
- implementing routine mediation with a social worker to update medical condition and healthcare decisions along every stage of the disease.

Chapter 31
Guardianship

A person's inability to remember, comprehend, and discern puts them at a higher risk of abuse. Family members can petition the court for guardianship if they suspect the person with Alzheimer's is being exploited, neglected, abused, or mistreated in any way.

My father named me as his guardian in his advanced directives if ever a court intervened in his care. But I didn't know a judge could overrule his decision. Marie tried for months to remove me and my brother from my father's life. I realize now how important it was to initiate mediation with Marie and her social worker to tell my side of the story. The result was that Marie had no legal justification to remove me as my father's advocate. And her quest to attain guardianship never succeeded.

However, there are family members and others whose concerns are valid, and their intentions and actions are honest and there are cases in which legal guardianship is necessary. My situation with Marie made me want to learn more about guardianship. I discovered that legal guardianships have been overused and infiltrated with corruption and abuse. Abusers are most often trusted individuals who are family members, caretakers, loved ones, advocates, and even legal guardians who work for the court system.

"Guardianship, also, referred to as conservatorship, is a legal process, utilized when a person can no longer make or communicate safe or sound decisions about his/her person and/or property or has become susceptible to fraud or undue influence. Because establishing a guardianship may remove considerable rights from an individual, it should only be considered after alternatives to guardianship have proven ineffective or are unavailable."[55] From the National Guardianship Association, "What Is Guardianship?"

The American Bar Association reports, "The legal system admits, problems exist in legal guardianships, but no one knows the true scope or what determinations the courts made in deciding a guardian was needed. They don't know who the guardians are, or what reports show or are being filed. Neither are they aware of how many questions or complaints against guardians have been raised with the courts. Without technical assistance and funding most under-resourced courts systems are unable to collect data. The result is we know there are problems, but we have no idea the true scope."[56] From the American Bar Association, "Challenges in Guardianship and Guardianship Abuse."

Guardianships are intended to protect the incapacitated, like my father. Yet, the reality is, that the courts are unable to track and monitor the guardians they have appointed. It's no wonder the system has become a magnet and a haven for predators. The American Bar Association's research into guardianship revealed. "Silver Collar Crimes" are financially motivated crimes intentionally perpetrated against elder persons with diminished cognition, using the court system or legal documents. Schemes occasionally involve unreasonably separating incapacitated persons from family, and misusing medications and drugs. There is a need for training of judges, lawyers, and court personnel on protecting due process rights in guardianship and conservatorship cases."[57] From the American Bar Association, "Uncovering Guardianship Abuse."

We can't wait for more funding, education, and training for judges, lawyers, and court personnel. By the time the system figures out how to track its guardians and the people they are supposed to be protecting how many will be exploited, abused, and neglected? The truth is no one knows.

Chapter 32
Why Lucidity is Important

During my father's Alzheimer's, I doubted the glimpses of awareness he had. For example, when he said to Marie, *Didn't we just get a check?* His memory was triggered by the commercial on the television. I didn't read into his comment because I wasn't aware that triggers can increase mental clarity. There were other moments, like the day of my stepson Danny's graduation party. My father's spontaneous awareness that he had Alzheimer's had occurred out of nowhere.

Researchers are learning more about lucid moments and the information I found has made me rethink one event in particular. It was late fall of 2017, before my father's lung cancer diagnosis. He and Marie were getting ready to leave my house after staying over for the weekend. It was their last visit before heading to Florida. My father wore his coat and a Scally hat and we were standing at the cellar door in the kitchen. He hugged me goodbye, held on, and said, "I don't want to go into a home. Please, don't put me in one."

Marie was in the kitchen with us. She didn't make a sound. I paid no attention to her non-reaction. This fear was lodged in his psyche for decades. I thought it was his Alzheimer's talking.

I said, "You're not going to a home, Dad."

Mark and I walked him and Marie to the car like always. We hugged again and my father got into the passenger seat. He stared at me, and his eyes filled up. He waved and didn't take his eyes off me as they pulled away. Our goodbye never felt so sad. He was aware and his fears were real.

Understanding the temporal lobe will help you to understand moments of clarity and lucid episodes. "The temporal lobe is a part of your brain that helps you use your senses to understand and respond to the world around you. It also plays a key role in how you communicate with other people, your ability to access memories, use language, and process emotions."[58] From the Cleveland Clinic, "Temporal Lobe: What It Is, Function, Location & Damage."

"There are several distinct types of lucid episodes one of which is called stimulus-induced lucidity. Researchers have discovered that in these episodes lucid moments are triggered by specific external stimuli, such as familiar music, faces, or environmental cues. These stimuli appear to evoke memories or emotions, temporarily lifting the veil of cognitive impairment and facilitating clearer communication and engagement."[59]

The other types of lucidity include:

"*Spontaneous Lucidity*—These are instances where individuals experience heightened moments of clarity that are not linked to any person, place, or thing that triggers their episode. Despite these unpredictable episodes, they offer valuable insights into the potential for short-term improvements in the thinking and reasoning abilities among people living with Alzheimer's and related dementias."[60]

The importance of social interactions with loved ones and connecting with friends can't be overstated.

"*Caregiver-Induced Lucidity*—These episodes are brought about by interactions with caregivers or loved ones. Personal connections and familiar interactions can enable a person to have a moment of clarity. These connections and interactions contribute to increased cognitive function. This underscores the profound positive impact of social support."[61]

"*Time-Bound Lucidity*—These are lucid episodes that occur consistently at specific times of the day or in relation to daily routines. These episodes of processing and retrieving information suggest there is a potential 24-hour cycle or environmental influence on cognitive function. This highlights the importance of routine and structure in supporting cognitive health."[62]

"*Sleep-Related Lucidity*—Instances of lucidity occurring during sleep or upon awakening. Despite disruptions in sleep patterns commonly experienced by individuals with advanced dementia, some may exhibit brief periods of clarity during these transitions, offering a fascinating glimpse into the interplay between sleep and cognitive function."[63] From LTC News, "Exploring Lucid Episodes in Late-Stage Alzheimer's Disease and Related Dementias."

Chapter 33
Types of Abuse

Our attorney didn't believe me when I expressed my suspicions of abuse while he was living alone with Marie. This leads me to believe that other family members aren't always taken seriously when they express their suspicions against another family member. The fact is, coercion, intimidation, and threats against a person with Alzheimer's are difficult to detect and harder to prove.

    A thirty-second commercial aimed at educating the public on elder abuse, or a webpage highlighting the warning signs of emotional torment, and exploitation with bullet points doesn't give family members and advocates effective strategies to prevent abuse against our most vulnerable population.

    I didn't believe my father's fear of going into a nursing home had anything to do with Marie. I accused Alzheimer's disease, instead of listening to what he said and asking more questions as to why he brought it up. I thought this fear was coming from him. However, after researching lucidity and Alzheimer's, I studied the situation again. I looked at the timing of my father's fear, his awareness, and his raw emotional state. This led me to believe that an active threat was looming over him and a trigger was involved. There was a stimulus that reinforced my father's fears and triggered his plea not to be admitted into a care home before he left that weekend. Marie's behavioral pattern of silence and non-reaction while my father emotionally unraveled was a clue as to who triggered it.

    A person who intentionally instills fear to threaten and control another person's actions and what they say is committing abuse.

Types of Abuse

Emotional torment and isolation leave no trail when there are no witnesses or evidence. These crimes become invisible and prosecuting the abuser is nearly impossible when the victim can't remember, or they are too afraid to speak out.

The first step in preventing abuse is to spot it. I discovered there are distinct types of abuse.

Coercive Control

What are the chances an attorney, or a physician, will mistake an abuser who is accompanying their client/patient, for the loving caretaker they portray themselves to be?

"Coercive control is a form of elder abuse. People who wish to influence or manipulate an older family member for their own benefit will often use coercive control to do so under the cover of 'simply providing care'. It's a type of abuse that often starts slowly but increases over time, and it is frequently mixed with loving and conciliatory behavior from the perpetrator. This inconsistency, and the fact that it does not always involve physical violence, means coercive control can be difficult to recognize and very difficult to prove."[64] From Compass Guiding Action on Elder Abuse. "Understanding Coercive Control as Elder Abuse."

Isolation

Marie physically separated my father from me, and my brother. She enraged him and tried to make him break off his relationship with us. Then Marie tried to keep him in Florida at the end of his life. She manipulated a rift in his friendship with Murray and blamed it on my father. Marie stopped taking my father to the social events they both once frequented at the clubhouse in their Florida condo community. She monitored every call he made. I believe she did it because she feared the unpredictable lucid moments. Now, I wonder if there were times when my father wanted to call me but didn't. "The abuser monitors and controls the victim's communication and interactions with others, including phone calls, messages, and social media. The victim becomes increasingly isolated from friends, family, and other social connections."[65]

Threats

"Intimidation is a way to prevent a victim from taking action against an abuser, and the threats can come in a variety of forms. The abuser uses threats of harm, violence, or other consequences to control the victim. Because of that, the victim feels fear or anxiety due to the abuser's threats or aggressive behavior."[66]

Gaslighting

"Gaslighting is a form of manipulation. It's a tactic in which someone claims that reality is different from how the victim is perceiving it. The abuser distorts the victim's perception of reality, making them doubt their memory, feelings, or sanity."[67] From Verywell Mind, "Look Out for These 4 Early Signs of Coercive Control."

Covert Abuse

"Covert abuse can apply to all types of cruelty, manipulation, and harm inflicted on another person. This isolation may be extreme, such as moving a person to a new town or city, with no nearby friends, relatives, or allies. It may also be less conspicuous, a suggestion that the individual's family and friends don't actually want to be around them. Covert abuse is rarely (if ever) a one-time occurrence but is often an ongoing, regular series of pain and distress for the individual being abused. Domestic violence perpetrators typically select partners, friends, or others close to them who will not stand up to abuse, to keep themselves in a place of power. Covert abuse frequently relies on the destabilization of the person who is being abused."[68] From Betterhelp, "Signs of Covert Abuse."

How Do You Stop Abuse That You Suspect?

- An investigation takes time. Therefore, I suggest you begin the investigation by contacting your social worker who you have been using from the beginning of the disease. They can help you file a report.
- "Adult Protective Services will determine if your report meets the state's criteria to open an investigation."[69]

- "If the individual you're concerned about is in immediate danger, call 911. If you only suspect abuse and haven't witnessed it firsthand, it may not get a police response. Sometimes a police presence can place individuals with certain disabilities in additional danger. If they react impulsively or are unable to communicate to police regarding what happened, or have acted in self-defense, the situation can escalate."[70] From DomesticShelters.org, "A Guide to Domestic Violence and Disabilities."
- If you suspect a hired caretaker of abuse, call their supervisor immediately, and file a formal complaint with their company or organization.

Mediate. Separate. Initiate.

- I suggest immediate intervention through mediation if you suspect abuse by a family member, who either lives with the person or visits regularly.
- Separate the suspect from the person with Alzheimer's.
- Initiate supervised visits only.
- Don't wait. Abuse is difficult to detect, and it takes time to prove.
- Do not attempt to handle this on your own.

Record, Document, and Communicate

During mediation with a social worker:

- Stay composed.
- Call out the behavior and actions.
- Decipher facts.
- I suggest allowing the person with Alzheimer's to attend part of this mediation if they are able.
- Watch their body language. Listen to what they say.

Chapter 34

How to Protect Against Financial Exploitation

How can we protect our loved ones with Alzheimer's from family predators and strangers who want to exploit their mental impairment? I suggest you begin securing the person's finances as soon as a diagnosis is made.

"Financial exploitation refers to two types of financial crimes committed against older adults. Financial abuse is committed by someone you know. Financial fraud is committed by a stranger. Both result in serious financial, physical, and emotional harm to older adults."[71] From the US Department of Justice, Elder Justice Initiative, "Financial Exploitation."

How to secure finances:

- Stop the use of ATMs and debit cards by the person with Alzheimer's.

- For the person's credit cards, close all but one. Set a charge limit. Call the number on the back of the credit card to disable cash advance. If the credit card does not have this option, limit cash advance to the lowest amount possible.

- Stop access by multiple family members and caretakers to cash, credit cards, and financial accounts. I recommend including the social worker for this discussion with family members, and caretakers.

- If the person with Alzheimer's needs money daily, I suggest they use their one credit card with a preset charge limit. Monitor it and pay it off monthly to keep the charge limit low.
- The financial power of attorney should be the only one with access to debit cards, checking/savings accounts, and investments and retirement accounts.
- Ask for receipts for incurred expenses like groceries, prescriptions, medical supplies, and gas to get to and from medical appointments.
- Set up a payment schedule with family caregivers, if you don't want to pay immediately upon receiving the receipt.
- Check in with the social worker at follow-up meetings. When people don't feel trusted, it can fuel resentment. I suggest you have the social worker reaffirm these steps are taken to protect the person with Alzheimer's from financial loss. This is a security strategy. It's not intended to hurt people's feelings.

Credit Freeze

As another layer of security, I suggest a credit freeze.

Contact each of the three credit bureaus to request:
- a fraud alert
- a credit freeze
- and a request a copy of the credit report and check for unusual activity.

The Federal Trade Commission's Consumer Information: www.consumer.ftc.gov

The only free source to access free credit reports: https://www.annualcreditreport.com/requestReport/landingPage.action

Equifax 888-378-4329 equifax.com,

Experian 888-397-3742 experian.com,

TransUnion 800-916-8800 transunion.com.

"A credit freeze restricts access to your credit report, which means you — or others — won't be able to open a new credit account while the freeze is in place. A credit freeze is free. It lasts until you remove it."[72] According to the Federal Trade Commission's Consumer Advice, "Credit Freeze or Fraud Alert: What's Right for Your Credit Report?"

Fraud Alert

"A fraud alert on a credit report notifies potential lenders and credit companies that you could be a potential fraud victim. When you place a fraud alert on your credit report, you can get a free copy of your credit report from each of the three credit bureaus."[73]

- "Anyone who suspects fraud can place a fraud alert on their credit report."[74]
- Check the credit report for any suspicious activity. Look for any new accounts. When were they opened?
- "A fraud alert will make it harder for someone to open a new credit account in your name. Businesses must verify your identity before they issue new credit in your name."[75] From the Federal Trade Commission Consumer Advice, "What to Know About Credit Freezes and Fraud Alerts."

"With an initial one-year fraud alert, credit grantors are required to use reasonable procedures to verify your identity. If, as part of placing an initial fraud alert, you provide a telephone number, they are also encouraged to call you at that phone number as part of that verification process. This can make it more difficult for an identity thief or fraudster to open new accounts or modify some parts of an existing account in your name."[76] From the Equifax.com, "7 Things to Know About Fraud Alerts."

"Long before people develop dementia, they often begin falling behind on mortgage payments, credit card bills, and other financial obligations, new research shows. A team of economists and medical experts at the Federal Reserve Bank of New York and Georgetown University combined Medicare records with data from Equifax, the credit bureau, to study how people's borrowing behavior changed in the years before and after a diagnosis of Alzheimer's or a similar disorder. What they found was striking: Credit scores among people who later develop dementia begin falling sharply long before their disease is formally identified. A year before diagnosis, these people were 17.2 percent more likely to be delinquent on their mortgage payments than before the onset of the disease, and 34.3 percent more likely to be delinquent on their credit card bills. The issues start even earlier: The study finds evidence of people falling behind on their debts five years before diagnosis. Credit scores and delinquencies, consistently worsen over time as the diagnosis approaches, it literally mirrors the changes in cognitive decline that we're observing, said Carole Roan Gresenz, a Georgetown University economist who was one of the study's authors."[77] From New York Times, "Alzheimer's Takes a Financial Toll Long Before Diagnosis, Study Finds."

Banks

Theft can occur in plain sight. A person with Alzheimer's can cash a check standing in front of a bank teller and then hand over their money to another party. It's that easy. No force is needed.

- I advise power of attorney to be filed with the bank. Use online banking. And remove the need for the person to go to the bank.
- Request all bank accounts state: power of attorney, plus the power of attorney's name, together with the person with Alzheimer's name.
- A person with Alzheimer's should not be carrying a large amount of cash. My father liked to keep a roll of bills in his pocket. Marie regularly took him to the bank to withdraw funds from his checking account inside the bank with a teller and an ATM. I don't advise this.
- If the person with Alzheimer's does go to the bank regularly, I recommend the person with power of attorney contact the

bank manager and inform them of the person's Alzheimer's diagnosis. This creates a layer of security.
- I advise the person who is power of attorney to inform the manager of the direct deposit checks, such as Social Security, pension, IRAs, etc.
- Ask for the person's accounts to be flagged as high risk of theft due to Alzheimer's diagnosis.
- Request to be notified if there is an attempt to cash a check by the person with Alzheimer's. This is important because changing direct deposit to paper checks over the phone is easy.

Remember: Coercion can be as gentle as telling the Alzheimer's person to repeat what is said.
- I recommend that the person with power of attorney check in monthly with the bank manager.

Steps to Investigating a Financial Account

1. Request the history of the financial account going back before your loved one's diagnosis.
2. Establish the baseline. The normal pattern within the account
3. Divide the monthly financial statements into timelines by using the corresponding physician's evaluations for Alzheimer's.
4. Take the stacks and compare spending according to the timelines and cognitive function.
5. If you suspect theft, jot down answers to these questions:
    - Have there been any changes or updates made to personal contact information such as:
    - a new address, phone number, or email?
    - a change in fund distribution. i.e.: direct deposit to mailed paper checks?

How to Protect Against Financial Exploitation

- increase in distribution amounts?
- rollovers of funds into other accounts?

6. Take note of any life changes that occurred within the time in question. Examples:
    - Was the person dating? If so, who?
    - Was there a new marriage?
    - Did someone move in or out of the home?
    - Any major renovations in the home? If so, who had access to personal information?
    - Was there a physical move to a new residence? If so:
    - Who are the new friends?
    - Has a key to the home been given out recently?

Through the process of elimination, narrow down the threat. When you have evidence, submit it to the police. I urge you not to confront the person you suspect.

"Every year, millions of older Americans lose significant portions of their life savings to elder financial exploitation, and the problem is only growing. During the pandemic, the rate of exploitation doubled, and some pandemic-related forms of exploitation are here to stay. Elder financial exploitation (EFE) is 'the illegal or improper use of an older adult's funds, property, or assets.' Perpetrators range from family members and other people a victim knows. Through this kind of exploitation, many victims are stripped of a significant part of their retirement savings. Getting restitution is nearly impossible."[78] From AARP, "The Scope of Elder Financial Exploitation: What It Costs Victims."

- To deter abuse, be vigilant in mediation with a social worker to improve communication, increase transparency, and dissolve disputes among family members and advocates. Then with the social worker's assistance, educate advocates and family members on the signs of abuse and emotional harm.

People with Alzheimer's fall victim not only to predators and opportunists but also—in some instances, to the legal system. "Every day the lives of older adults are profoundly and negatively impacted in both the criminal and civil justice systems based on mistaken assumptions and inadequate assessments of their capacity to make decisions for themselves."[79] From the Elder Justice Symposium, United States Department of Justice, "Elder Justice Initiative."

Is an attorney's assessment of a client's ability to make decisions for themselves always accurate?

I discovered how difficult it is for an attorney to detect impaired judgment. Aimee Smith, an attorney who focuses her practice on issues related to elder law, wrote an article in Lawyer's Mutual, a liability insurance company whose job it is to help attorneys prevent claims. Smith states, "One of the trickiest, most subjective things we do as attorneys is assessing whether our clients have the requisite capacity to execute legal documents. As an elder law attorney, I regularly deal with clients who have diminished capacity for one reason or another. Diminished capacity is not always evident. This is particularly true if the client is a new client for whom you have no frame of reference."[80] From Lawyers Mutual Insurance Company, "Assessing the Legal Capacity of Our Clients."

Attorneys are human. That means they are fallible. This is why I urge advocates and family members to use a social worker as part of your care team. Use your three main tools: record, document, and communicate from the onset of diagnosis.

- Listen carefully and watch the body language of the person with Alzheimer's and the people who surround them.
- Empower yourselves through knowledge.
- Our loved ones with Alzheimer's are depending on us. We can protect them.

In Closing

I want to take you to August 1, 1998. Day 48. My father's last day of the Big Ride Across America.

> *51.4 miles left.*
> *Leaving Frederick MD and pedaling into Washington DC.*
>
> *It's our final day. The hills and mountains are behind us. It's my first day that I haven't had any pain in my legs. I feel tremendous. Mike and I were riding together, and I just feel like letting it all hang out. I came out of the saddle and rode like I never had before. Greg LeMond couldn't have come near me. I passed every bike for the next twenty miles. I was flying. I just felt so great not to have any pain. The traffic was real heavy and again we kept our fingers crossed and as we rode into the holding area and the people were cheering and clapping. I said we made it. That's all I cared about and I put my hand on Sis's picture, and I said a prayer. I knew she was with me all the time. I could feel it. I can't wait to see Jacqueline and John and Marie. Although, I won't see John until I get home. Then someone put their hands over my eyes. I didn't know who it was. Sure enough, it was Jacqueline. What a sight to see her and then John. I missed them terribly. It was so good to see them and then Marie. She looked great. I was so happy to have made it. For five years I wanted to do this and now it's done but it's not over. Not until a cure is found for cancer. The disease does not rest, and neither will I. There will be more rides and walks till we bury this disease once and for all.*

Fear Knocked — Jacqueline Sullivan Wyco

For my father, there was no challenge too big that he didn't strive to overcome. He was one ordinary man who left the people he touched with an extraordinary sense of what it means to be a great man and a good person.

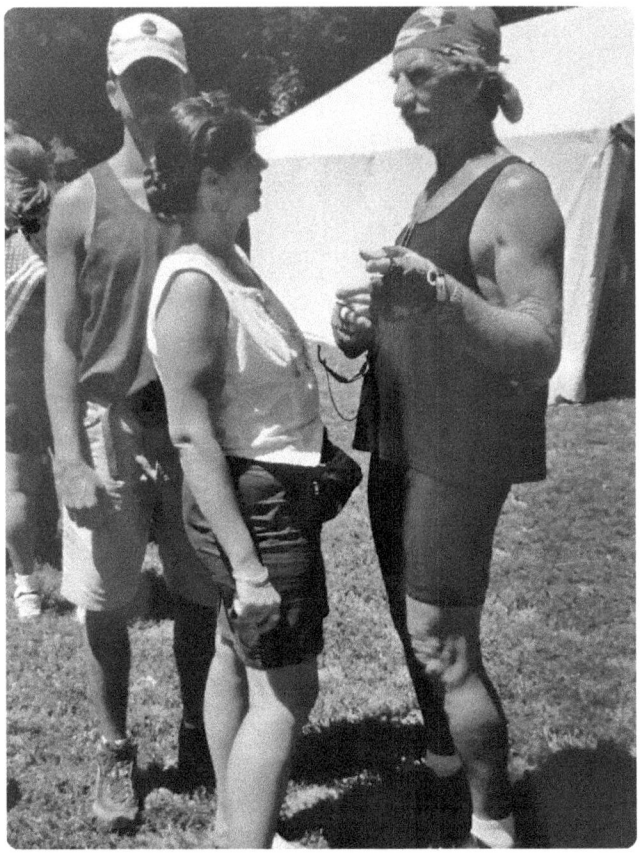

Author Jacqueline in the front. Back left is John, her brother, and her father, to the right. *Photographer unknown, from the Sullivan Family Photo Collection*

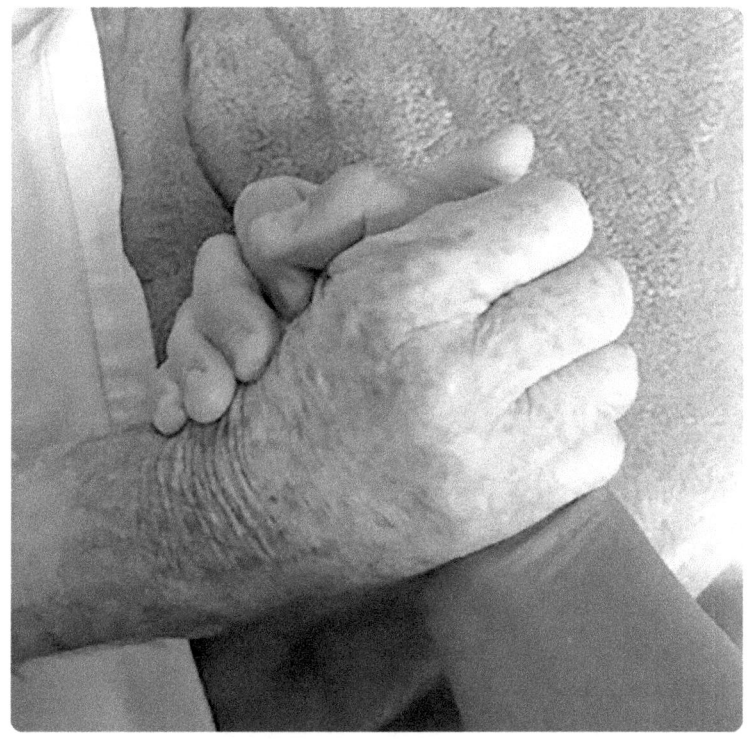
Author's brother holding their father's hand on September 11, 2018, 2 days before he died. *From the Sullivan Family Photo Collection*

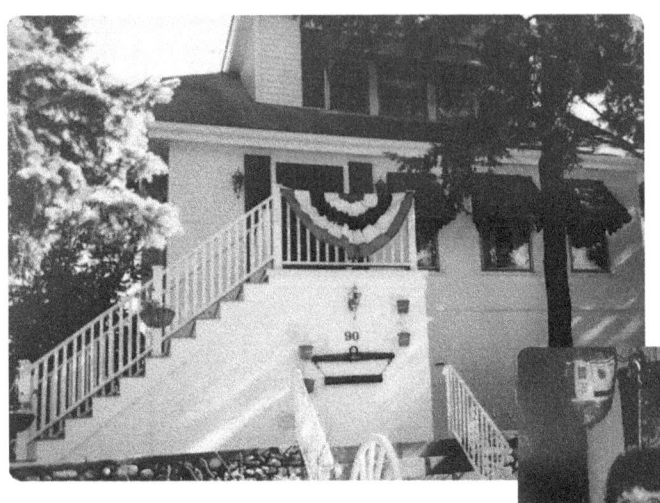

Sullivan family home in 2010. *All photos on this page are from the Sullivan Family photo collection.*

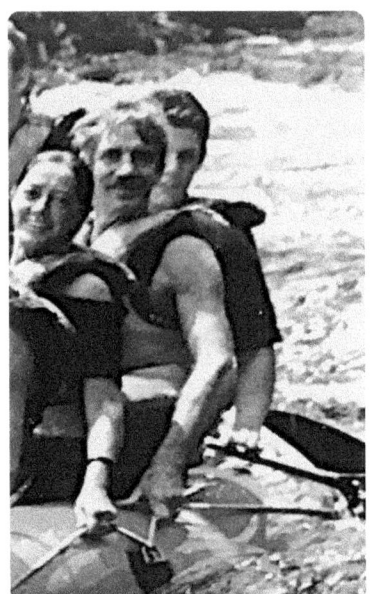

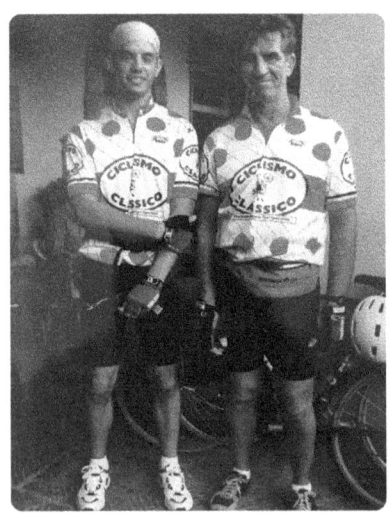

Above, Jacqueline's mother Beverly (Sis), her father (Sully), John, and her brother John on a river rapids ride about 1987.

Above right, Jacqueline and her father in his kitchen on Thanksgiving Day 1998.

At right, 1994 Jacqueline's brother John and their father on the cycling trip in Italy he won in a raffle his first year riding the Pan Mass Challenge.

Obituary
John "Jack" Sullivan, Jr.

John "Jack" Sullivan Jr., 79, formerly of West Roxbury died on Thursday, September 13, 2018, at a Hospice House in Worcester, MA, surrounded by his family. He was born in Jamaica Plain, Boston to John J. and Mary (Molly) T. (McCarthy) Sullivan.

No matter how many times Jack got knocked down, he got up twice as many. Jack fought hard as hell to stay. Alzheimer's and lung cancer couldn't keep Jack from wanting to live. He had the strength, stability, and determination of an ox. https://www.milesfuneralhome.com/obituaries/John-Jack-Sullivan-2/#!/obituary

Jack's life, first and foremost, was centered around his family. He always said, "There's nothing like family." He was there whenever we needed him. There was nothing he wouldn't do for us. He was kind, generous, hardworking, honest, and full of pride and integrity. Jack lived his life every day with optimism. He brought happiness to each and every person, every day. He was always helping others.

Jack proudly served in the United States Marine Corps. And afterwards, went on to work in Local 534 Boston Plasterers and Cement Masons Union for more than 35 years. He used to joke and say that Boston was his city because he helped build it, which he did. He worked on all the major buildings in the 1960s through the early 1990s like the Prudential, The John Hancock, The Marriot Long Wharf, The Westin at Copley Place, The Ted Williams Tunnel; you name it, he most likely worked on it. He worked sometimes round the clock, pouring and finishing concrete. He loved Boston.

In 1973, Jack became a Boston Firefighter. He was first stationed in Brighton at Oak Square. He transferred to Ladder 7 at Meetinghouse

Hill in Dorchester, MA. because he wanted to be at a busier house, and a busier house he surely got. Ladder 7 during the 1970s and early 1980s was literally blazing. A June 16, 1982, New York Times headline read "Boston Is Becoming the Hub of Arson." Jack was fearless. At one point in time, Ladder 7 was one of the busiest firehouses in the nation.

Jack worked both jobs his entire career. He loved them both. He loved the guys, he always said, "They were good guys." He loved to laugh and joke around.

Every summer Jack took his family camping. He took his family all over the place, from salmon fishing on Lake Ontario in New York to one of his favorite places, Scusset Beach, Cape Cod. He loved to fish and was self-taught. Every spring he would stop at Jamaica Pond on the way to work to throw a few casts in to catch trout. In the winter he ice-fished. In the summer, he fished in the Cape Cod Canal with his son John. In his earlier days, he hunted. He loved being outdoors. Jack took pride in his home and spent countless hours working outside landscaping and gardening.

After his first wife, Beverly "Sis," died of cancer in 1992, Jack began another journey. He took his grief and poured it into raising money to help find a cure for cancer. In 1993 he started riding the Pan Mass Challenge. A 192-mile bike ride from Sturbridge to Provincetown over the course of one weekend. He loved it. He did this for many years. When he was 59 years old, he decided to do even more. He entered The Big Ride, a six-and-a-half week, 3,300-mile ride from Seattle, Washington to Washington, DC for American Lung Cancer. In the months leading up to the ride, he trained relentlessly. On The Big Ride, he endured all kinds of weather. One day the weather was so bad at Mount Helena that the support vehicle picked up all the riders and brought them to the next base camp for that night. The next morning Jack got up, found a rancher, and paid him to bring him back to the spot where he was picked up the day before. Jack wanted to make sure he pedaled every step of the way. He did 130 miles just on that day; Jack made lifelong friends on that trip. Jack raised $10,000 alone for American Lung Cancer that year and many thousands for the Pan-Mass Challenge over the years.

In 2013, Jack married Marie. They met ballroom dancing in 1998

Obituary: John "Jack" Sullivan, Jr.

and shared 21 years together. They enjoyed Florida in the winter and Cape Cod in the summer. They enjoyed life. Together they ballroom danced, went to the beach, dined out, and traveled all over Europe and the United States. They were always on the go. They lived life to the fullest. Jack was a magnet. Everywhere he went people were drawn to him. He knew everyone. It didn't matter where he was, he would always bump into someone he knew. He loved people; he loved to make them laugh.

Jack was also notorious for being lucky. People he knew would actually rub his arm, hoping that some of his luck would rub off on them. If you were at any event that had a raffle, you could bet money that Jack would win something. One year he won the raffle at The Pan Mass Challenge. He won a trip for two to cycle through Italy which he and his son did. He did have a little luck of the Irish.

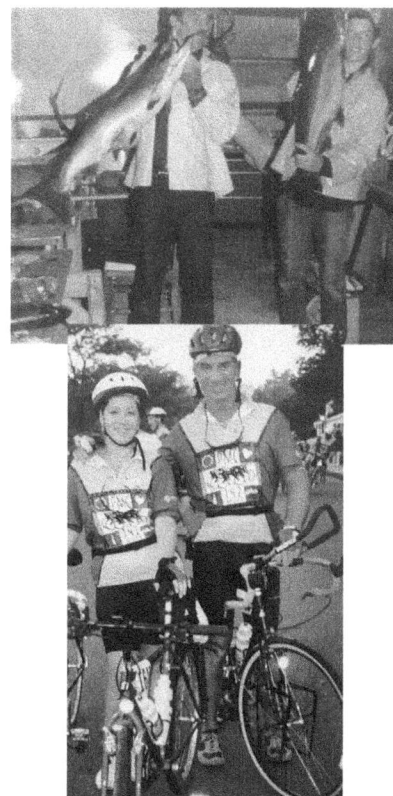

Jacqueline and her father
1995 Pan Mass Challenge

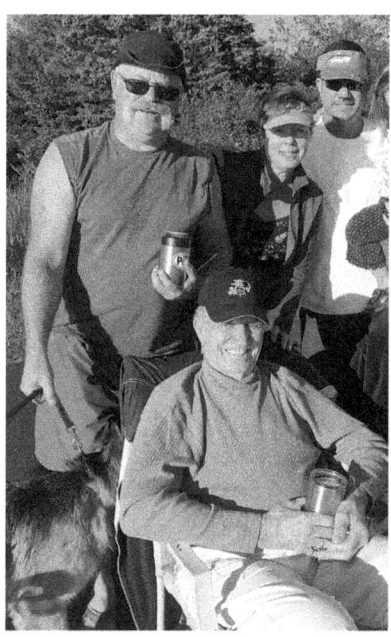

At left, Jacqueline's father and her brother John salmon fishing at Lake Ontario, New York in 1989.

Left to right Jacqueline's husband Mark, Jacqueline, her brother John, his daughter Beverly, and her father in the front. Cape Cod Canal October 1, 2017.

Endnotes

Chapter 1

1. "Time Period: The Great Depression | Federal Reserve History," n.d. *https://www.federalreservehistory.org/time-period/great-depression*

2. Bing. "Mather Elementary - Bing," n.d. *https://www.bing.com/search?q=mather+elementary*

3. Wikipedia contributors. "Boston Desegregation Busing Crisis." Wikipedia, March 12, 2025. *https://en.wikipedia.org/wiki/Boston_desegregation_busing_crisis*

Chapter 2

4. 5. 6. 7. Marina Manoukian, "The Untold Truth Behind the 1982 Boston Arson Spree," Grunge, February 16, 2022, *https://www.grunge.com/769980/the-untold-truth-behind-the-1982-boston-arson-spree/*

8. "Amazon.com : Burn Boston Burn Book," n.d. *https://www.amazon.com/s?k=burn+boston+burn+book&crid=2ME0MV968OL2O&sprefix=burn+boston+burn 2Caps%2C137&ref=nb_sb_ss_ts-doa-p_3_16*

9. "1982 Boston Arson Spree." Wikipedia. August 2, 2023. *https://en.wikipedia.org/wiki/1982_Boston_arson_spree*

Chapter 4

10. Mayo Clinic. "Alzheimer's Stages: How the Disease Progresses," n.d. *https://www.mayoclinic.org/diseases-conditions/alzheimers-disease/in-depth/alzheimers-stages/art-20048448*

Chapter 5

11. Archana Gaur, Ariyanachi Kaliappan, Yuvaraj Balan, Varatharajan Sakthivadivel, Kalpana Medala, and Madhusudhan Umesh, "Sleep and Alzheimer: The Link," March 17, 2022, https://doi.org/10.26574/maedica.2022.17.1.177

12. 13. 14. Nam-Gyoon Kim, and Ho-Won Lee, "Stereoscopic Depth Perception and Visuospatial Dysfunction in Alzheimer's Disease," Healthcare, February 3, 2021, https://doi.org/10.3390/healthcare9020157

15. Mayo Clinic. "Learn How Alzheimer's Is Diagnosed," n.d. https://www.mayoclinic.org/diseases-conditions/alzheimers-disease/in-depth/alzheimers/art-20048075

Chapter 6

16. Csn, Amy Isler Rn, Msn,. "Losing Your Sense of Smell May Be a Warning Sign of Alzheimer's." Verywell Health, August 15, 2023. https://www.verywellhealth.com/losing-sense-of-smell-alzheimers-early-sign-7642332

17. Aria Jafari, Laura de Lima Xavier, Jeffrey D. Bernstein, Kristina Simonyan, and Benjamin S. Bleier, "Association of Sinonasal Inflammation with Functional Brain Connectivity," National Library of Medicine, June 1, 2021, https://pubmed.ncbi.nlm.nih.gov/33830194/

18. Huaxiong Zhang, Yiya Zhang, Yangfan Li, Yaling Wang, Sha Yan, San Xu, Zhili Deng, Xinling Yang, Hongfu Xie, and Ji Li, "Bioinformatics and Network Pharmacology Identify the Therapeutic Role and Potential Mechanism of Melatonin in AD and Rosacea," National Library of Medicine, November 23, 2012, https://www.ncbi.nlm.nih.gov/pmc/articles/pmc8657413/

19. Fen-Fang Hong, Shu-Long Yang, Huang Kuang, Yu-Ge Zhu, Zhi-Feng Zhou, and Mei-Wen Yang, "Sleep Disorders in Alzheimer's Disease: The Predictive Roles and Potential Mechanisms," National Library of Medicine, October 16, 2021, https://pubmed.ncbi.nlm.nih.gov/33642368/

20. 21. Leslie Kernisan MD MPH, "Financial Exploitation in Aging: What to Know & What to Do," Better Health While Aging, July 27, 2018, https://betterhealthwhileaging.net/financial-abuse-what-to-know/

Chapter 8

22. "Swiss Cheese Model." Wikipedia. Wikimedia Foundation. March 29, 2019, https://en.wikipedia.org/wiki/Swiss_cheese_model

Chapter 9

23. 24. Lamothe, Cindy. "How to Recognize Coercive Control." Healthline, October 10, 2019. https://www.healthline.com/health/coercive-control

25. Professional, Cleveland Clinic Medical. "Sundown Syndrome." Cleveland Clinic, March 19, 2025. https://my.cleveland-clinic.org/health/articles/22840-sundown-syndrome

Chapter 10

26. Vantage Point Consulting. "De-escalation and Calming Techniques for Dementia Sufferers." Vantage Point Consulting (blog), July 12, 2022. https://vantagepointc.com/de-escalation-and-calming-techniques-for-dementia-sufferers/

27. Professional, Cleveland Clinic Medical. "Sundown Syndrome." Cleveland Clinic, March 19, 2025. https://my.cleveland-clinic.org/health/articles/22840-sundown-syndrome

Chapter 11

28. Crystal Gwizdala, "When Personal and Professional Morals Clash: Conscientious Objection in Medicine," Yale School of Medicine, July 18, 2022, https://medicine.yale.edu/news-article/when-personal-and-professional-morals-clash-conscientious-objection-in-medicine/

29. "Law Notes." National Association of Social Workers. 2019. https://www.socialworkers.org/About/Legal/law-notes

Chapter 12

30. Shroeder, Becca. "Coercive Control: Abuse Hidden in Plain Sight." Domestic Violence Network, February 12, 2024. https://mgaleg.maryland.gov/cmte_testimony/2024/jud/1dn8POpod3i-FuKdmkHzbJtaPHecKUKd.pdf

Chapter 15

31. Ariane Resnick, "Look out for These 4 Early Signs of Coercive Control," Verywell Mind, January 2, 2024, https://www.verywellmind.com/early-signs-of-coercive-control-7963438

Chapter 16

32. Ariane Resnick, "Look out for These 4 Early Signs of Coercive Control," Verywell Mind, January 2, 2024, https://www.verywellmind.com/early-signs-of-coercive-control-7963438

Chapter 17

33. Rebecca Zerk, and Sarah Wydall. "The Combination of Dementia and Domestic Abuse Is All Too Often Overlooked," The Conversation, August 19, 2020, https://theconversation.com/the-combination-of-dementia-and-domestic-abuse-is-all-too-often-overlooked-139535

34. "Get the Facts on Elder Abuse." National Council on Aging. February 23, 2021. https://www.ncoa.org/article/get-the-facts-on-elder-abuse

Chapter 19

35, 36, 37. 38. 39 Winegarden, Jennifer, DO. "Dementia-related Pain: What Caregivers Need to Know." Mayo Clinic Health System, September 7, 2023.
https://www.mayoclinichealthsystem.org/hometown-health/speaking-of-health/dementia-related-pain-and-caregivers

Chapter 20

40. "The Combination of Dementia and Domestic Abuse Is All Too Often Overlooked." The Conversation, n.d. *https://theconversation.com/the-combination-of-dementia-and-domestic-abuse-is-all-too-often-overlooked-139535*

41. "Understanding Coercive Control as Elder Abuse." Compass Guiding Action on Elder Abuse. July 14, 2024. *https://www.compass.info/featured-topics/coercive-control/understanding-coercive-control-as-elder-abuse/#section-what-is-coercive-control*

Chapter 21

42. Morrow, Angela, RN. "Understanding and Recognizing Terminal Restlessness." Verywell Health, May 8, 2023. *https://www.verywellhealth.com/terminal-restlessness-1132271*

43. Aaron. "Hospice Pain Management: A Comprehensive Guide." Continua Learning, November 1, 2024. *https://continuagroup.com/article/hospice-pain-management/*

Chapter 22

44. Coyne, Patrick, Sarah Lowry, Carol Mulvenon, and Judith A. Paice. "American Society for Pain Management Nursing and Hospice and Palliative Nurses Association Position Statement: Pain Management at the End of Life." Pain Management Nursing 25, no. 4 (May 1, 2024): 327–29. *https://doi.org/10.1016/j.pmn.2024.03.020*

Chapter 23

45. Kinard, Jordan. "Why Dying People Often Experience a Burst of Lucidity." Scientific American, February 20, 2024. *https://www.scientificamerican.com/article/why-dying-people-often-experience-a-burst-of-lucidity/*

Chapter 24

46.47. Coyne, Patrick, Carol Mulvenon, and Judith A. Paice. "American Society for Pain Management Nursing and Hospice and Palliative Nurses Association Position Statement: Pain Management at the End of Life." Pain Management Nursing 19, no. 1 (December 16, 2017): 3–7. *https://doi.org/10.1016/j.pmn.2017.10.019*

Chapter 25

48. Mail, HelloCare. "Two-hourly Repositioning to Prevent Bedsores Is 'Abuse', Study Says.." Hellocare, February 2, 2021. *https://hellocare.com.au/two-hourly-repositioning-prevent-bedsores-abuse-study/*

Chapter 28

49, 50. Office of Inspector General | Government Oversight | U.S. Department of Health and Human Services. "Vulnerabilities in the Medicare Hospice Program Affect Quality Care and Program Integrity: An OIG Portfolio," February 27, 2024. *https://oig.hhs.gov/reports/all/2018/vulnerabilities-in-the-medicare-hospice-program-affect-quality-care-and-program-integrity-an-oig-portfolio/*

51. "Medicare Program; FY 2018 Hospice Wage Index and Payment Rate Update and Hospice Quality Reporting Requirements." Journal-article. Federal Register. Vol. 82, May 3, 2017. *https://www.govinfo.gov/content/pkg/FR-2017-05-03/pdf/2017-08563.pdf*

Chapter 30

52. Malkin, Craig, PhD. "Meet the Personality Type Most Prone to Secret Abuse." Psychology Today, February 16, 2018. *https://www.psychologytoday.com/us/blog/romance-redux/201802/what-everyone-should-know-about-covert-abusers?msockid=108744ba8ad0629308544a438b00633b*

53. Hall, Julie L. "Triangulating, Flattering, and Conducting Smear Campaigns." Psychology Today, September 10, 2023. *https://www.psychologytoday.com/us/blog/the-narcissist-in-your-life/202007/52-ways-to-identify-a-covert-narcissist?msockid=108744ba8ad0629308544a438b00633b*

54. Compassion & Choices. "Advance Care Planning - Compassion & Choices," n.d. *https://compassionandchoices.org/our-issues/advance-care-planning/*

Chapter 31

55. "What Is Guardianship?" National Guardianship Association. 2024. *https://www.guardianship.org/what-is-guardianship/*

56. Godfrey, David. "Challenges in Guardianship and Guardianship Abuse." ABA, March 11, 2021. *https://www.americanbar.org/groups/law_aging/publications/bifocal/vol-42/vol-42-issue-4-march-april-2021/challenges-in-guardianship-and-guardianship-abuse/*

57. Palmieri, Anthony. "Uncovering Guardianship Abuse." ABA, October 27, 2021. *https://www.americanbar.org/groups/senior_lawyers/resources/voice-of-experience/2010-2022/uncovering-guardianship-abuse/*

Chapter 32

58. Temporal Lobe." Cleveland Clinic, March 19, 2025. *https://my.clevelandclinic.org/health/body/16799-temporal-lobe*

59. 60. 61. 62. 63. James Kelly, Exploring Lucid Episodes in Late-Stage Alzheimer's Disease and Related Dementias, March 7, 2024, LTC News, *https://www.ltcnews.com/articles/lucid-episodes-alzheimers#:~:text=1%20Spontaneous%20Lucidity%3A%20These%20are%20instances%20where%20individuals*

Chapter 33

64. "Understanding Coercive Control as Elder Abuse." Compass Guiding Action on Elder Abuse. March 8, 2024. *https://www.compass.info/featured-topics/coercive-control/understanding-coercive-control-as-elder-abuse/#section-examples-of-coercive-control*

65. 66. 67. Cnc, Ariane Resnick. "4 Early Signs of Coercive Control." Verywell Mind, January 3, 2024. *https://www.verywellmind.com/early-signs-of-coercive-control-7963438*

68. BetterHelp Editorial Team. "Signs of Covert Abuse | BetterHelp," March 19, 2025. *https://www.betterhelp.com/advice/abuse/am-i-the-victim-of-covert-abuse-learning-the-signs/*

69. 70. Kippert, Amanda. "A Guide to Domestic Violence and Disabilities." DomesticShelters.org, July 1, 2024. *https://www.domesticshelters.org/articles/identifying-abuse/a-guide-to-domestic-violence-and-disabilities*

Chapter 34

71. "Financial Exploitation." United States. Department of Justice. *https://www.justice.gov/elderjustice/financial-exploitation*

72. 73. 74. 75. Consumer Advice. "Credit Freeze or Fraud Alert: What's Right for Your Credit Report?," April 10, 2025. *https://consumer.ftc.gov/articles/credit-freeze-or-fraud-alert-whats-right-your-credit-report*

76. Equifax. "7 Things to Know About Fraud Alerts." Equifax, 2023. *https://www.equifax.com/personal/education/identity-theft/articles/-/learn/7-things-to-know-about-fraud-alerts/*

77. Casselman, Ben. "Alzheimer's Takes a Financial Toll Long Before Diagnosis, Study Finds." New York Times, May 31, 2024. *https://www.nytimes.com/2024/05/31/business/economy/alzheimers-disease-personal-finance.html*

78. Gunther, Jilenne. "The Scope of Elder Financial Exploitation: What It Costs Victims." AARP, June 27, 2023. *https://www.aarp.org/pri/topics/work-finances-retirement/fraud-consumer-protection/scope-elder-financial-exploitation/?msockid=108744ba8ad0629308544a438b00633b*

79. "Elder Justice Initiative, Elder Justice Decision-Making Capacity Symposium," United States Department of Justice. February 23, 2022. *https://www.justice.gov/elderjustice/elder-justice-decision-making-capacity-symposium*

80. Lawyers Mutual Insurance of North Carolina. "Assessing the Legal Capacity of Our Clients - Lawyers Mutual Insurance NC," December 16, 2015. *https://lawyersmutualnc.com/article/assessing-the-legal-capacity-of-our-clients/*

Bibliography

Books
Caregiving

LeBlanc, Gary Joseph. *The Aftereffects of Caregiving*. 19 Aug. 2015.

LeBlanc, Gary Joseph. *Managing Alzheimer's and Dementia Behaviors (Health Care Edition)*. 13 Apr. 2016.

LeBlanc, Gary Joseph. *Staying Afloat in a Sea of Forgetfulness*. Xlibris Corporation, 2 June 2011.

LeBlanc, Gary Joseph. *Managing Alzheimer's and Dementia Behaviors*. 10 Nov. 2012.

Phelps, Rick. While I Still Can. Xlibris Corporation, 2012.

Guardianship

Sugar, Sam. *Guardianship and the Elderly: The Perfect Crime*. Garden City Park, NY, Square One Publishers, 2018.

Hackard, Michael. *The Wolf at the Door*. Hackard Global Media, 1 Nov. 2017.

Hackard, Michael. *Alzheimer's, Widowed Stepmothers & Estate Crimes*. 1 Mar. 2019.

Website Resources

Gary Joseph LeBlanc, Associate Executive Director for Dementia Spotlight Foundation *https://dementiaspotlightfoundation.org/gary-bio/*

Bill Brett. Link to his webpage to learn more about him, his photos and to purchase his books. https://billbrettboston.com/

Google George Rizer, photographer. He worked for The Boston Globe. His photos are dramatic. They pull you in and connect you to the time and place of the event he captured.

Assessment of Older Adults with Diminished Capacities 2nd Edition   This handbook is written by the American Bar Association Commission on Law and Aging American Psychological Association. It helped me to understand how attorneys determine whether a person like my father has the understanding and the ability to make legal documents. *https://www.apa.org/pi/aging/resources/guides/diminished-capacity.pdf*

Alzheimer's Association
https://www.alz.org

When Catherine Faulk's father, Peter Faulk, was in his final years of Alzheimer's disease she was banned from seeing him by her estranged stepmother. Her foundation seeks legislation across the country and provides resources for those who are trying to visit their parents after being denied.
https://catherinefaulkorganization.org/

Kerry Kasem, the daughter of Casey Kasem, addresses the experiences of an increasing number of families whose family members need protection from abuse, regardless of their financial status. Her webpage Kasem Cares promotes elder abuse awareness and education.
https://Kasemcares.org/

I found helpful information in the *Elder Justice Decision-Making Capacity Resource Guide* that explains the multiple misconceptions about decision-making capacity. *https://www.justice.gov*

Bibliography

The Centers for Medicare and Medicaid Services. Compare tools for doctors and clinicians. CMS.gov *https://www.cms.gov/medicare/quality/physician-compare-initiative*

Dr. Sam Sugar is a licensed physician and president of the Americans Against Abusive Probate Guardianship (AAAPG). His personal experience with the guardianship system led him to write and speak to expose the corruption and crimes committed against those who have been stripped of their rights, under legal guardianships. *https://www.injuredseniorpodcast.com/blog/how-to-prevent-guardianships-with-dr-sam-sugar/*

For First Responders in need of critical incident stress management, including pre-incident education, peer support, and debriefings, visit *https://onsiteacademy.org* "On-Site Academy is a short-term, intensive residential treatment center for rescue personnel who may be temporarily overwhelmed by the stress of their job, suffering from work-related cumulative or delayed critical incident stress, or experiencing an acute, transient reaction to a 'critical incident'."

Acknowledgments

To Mark Wyco, my husband, thank you for the care you gave my father in his last days at our home, and the support you gave him and me throughout his disease. Writing this book has consumed me for over six years. I want to thank you for giving me the space I needed to accomplish it.

Thank you to our son Danny, who is Worcester (MA) firefighter, and our daughter Kelsey, who is a 911 Police/Fire dispatcher for the City of Worcester, (MA), you have been kind and supportive of me since the day we met. And thank you to our daughter Sheila, who is a great mom to our two grandchildren, Alice and Liam.

To John, growing up, we were close. You are more than my brother. We are friends, and have been, our entire lives. We shared two amazing parents. Now, Beverly and Jack carry on their spirit.

To my sister-in-law, Karen, thank you for being there in the hospice and for the photos you took of Dad's helmet for his prayer card. The collages you made for his tribute showed who he was and how much he loved his family. Thank you for being a part of our family.

One teacher early on in my massage therapy training told me that each client who came to me seeking massage or energy work was a person I needed to learn from. The lessons I've learned throughout my life have extended to every meaningful working and personal relationship I've ever had. However brief or long my encounters have been, each person has taught me more about myself and my work than any book or study course I've ever taken.

To all the social workers of The Virginia Thurston Healing Garden Cancer Support Center where I worked for eleven years, specifically Brianne Carter, LICSW, Helene Gagliano, psychotherapist and medical counselor, and Marcia Lewin-Berlin, LICSW. Thank you for your support and guidance in my time there. My experience with all of you made me see that a social worker is essential for the security, protection, and overall well-being of a person with Alzheimer's.

To Courtney S., the social worker who helped me with Marie, thank you for being objective. You helped me when no one else did.

To Mike Keefe, my father lit up when he heard your name, and when he saw you, Joe Novelli, and the late George Piscitello, he remembered the bond you all shared. You have reinforced for me what it means to be a great friend.

To Mark Mathes, my editor, who took me on as a first-time author. Thank you for your expertise, professionalism, and guidance. Your honest comments, opinions, and questions have made my father's story one I am very proud of.

Thank you to Bill Brett, an award-winning photojournalist of The Boston Globe and a published author of six books. I emailed Bill and asked him if he could tell me who took the pictures of my father at fire scenes and accidents on the job back in the 1970s and 1980s. He emailed back *Call Me* with his number. When I spoke with Bill, I felt like I was talking with someone I knew. He referred me to George Rizer, another photographer for the Globe. Thank you, Bill.

To George Rizer, a Boston Globe photographer who captured the working lives of cops, fire, and EMS for forty years. I texted him and said Bill referred me. He replied and went through his files and sent me pictures that evening. He asked for nothing in return. Thank you so much, George.

Thank you to Haden Duggan, Ed.D., the president and founder of the On-Site Academy in Gardner, Massachusetts, a residential trauma treatment and training program for Public Safety Personnel, and grief counselor, Kathy Minehan. My husband Mark led the critical incidents stress team on the Worcester Fire Department. He reached out to Haden and Kathy for me. They helped me to piece back together my life after my father died. Thank you for the work you and your teams do.

To Maris Soule, an accomplished author I met in Florida, thank you for guiding me on traditional publishing and submissions.

Thank you to Nancy Koucky, of NRK Designs, whose expertise, attention to detail, and patience brought my vision onto the book cover and its content that hold my father's story.

Author's Note

Writing is cathartic, a form of healing. But I've got to tell you, along the way, it didn't always feel like that. Through this process, I am more convinced than ever that what I learned will help others.

For six years I focused on how I could have done better as an advocate. Why did I assume that my father's symptoms were that of normal aging and not Alzheimer's? It bothered me so much that I researched studies and made the connection to when his symptoms started.

I believed my father's second marriage was based on their mutual love for each other, family, and trust. What happened to him led me to learn more about detecting behavioral patterns associated with coercion and abuse.

Without justification, my father's physicians overrode his right to have me voice what he wanted for his own care. And then the unimaginable happened. When a hospice house failed to manage my father's pain at the end of his life, I wanted answers.

It took a lot of digging. But I put every piece of the aftermath back together. In doing so I saw the solutions to help others prevent a hospice nightmare.

I discovered that the laws, physicians, attorneys, guardianships, the courts, and advanced directives don't protect a person with Alzheimer's in the ways we think they do. Ultimately it is our responsibility to protect our parents, grandparents, and aging loved ones who are in decline. It's their right to have an advocate speak for them. You must strengthen their voice by using yours. They deserve to be heard. And their choices need to be protected.

—Jacqueline Sullivan Wyco, May 2025

About the Author

Jacqueline Sullivan Wyco is the author of *Fear Knocked*. Jacqueline lives in Venice, Florida with her husband Mark, a retired Worcester Fire Department Captain in Massachusetts.. Jacqueline was born and raised in Boston during the 1970s when violence exploded in the city and America's economy shifted into an all-out crisis. Her father, John Sullivan, fought fires and saved lives in the Dorchester neighborhood of Boston, during the largest arson case in history. In his second job as a union cement mason, he finished concrete during the construction of the most iconic buildings in Boston. The two jobs kept him away for days at a time. Her mother, Beverly Sullivan, stayed at home to raise her children. She filled both their roles while he was gone.

As a kid, Jacqueline remembered her father would begin the first phrase of the Irish proverb, *Fear knocked on the door*, then she'd answer with, *faith answered*, and they'd recite together, *and there was nobody there*. Her father instilled in her the belief that she could make it through anything, regardless of what life confronted her with.

Jacqueline cooked for thirty years, in every aspect of the business, from restaurants to country clubs, fine dining, catering, restaurants, independent living, and everything in between. Jacqueline worked as a chef and a manager for Boston's Hebrew Senior Life when the industry's priority shifted from the institutionalized nursing home culture to the new aging-in-place model of care. This concept brought forward what it meant to treat the most vulnerable with more compassion and understanding than ever before.

In 2008 Jacqueline embarked on a new career as a massage therapist and focused her business on the health and well-being of the aging. She reached out in her community in Cape Cod, Massachusetts to councils on aging, assisted living, and independent living centers where she provided an introductory presentation on the benefits of massage, and reiki. Twice a month in seven locations she provided these therapies. Her clients ranged in age, and many struggled with physical and cognitive challenges. Jacqueline believed knowledge was power, and she conducted ongoing workshops that engaged seniors and wrote newsletters to share what she thought could help them.

When Jacqueline married a Worcester firefighter, Mark Wyco, she moved and began her career in a new city. Jacqueline continued her education and trained to be an oncology massage therapist, manual lymphatic drainage practitioner, and reiki master/teacher. She provided these therapies to clients seeking to feel whole again. She discovered a non-profit organization that provided all types of therapeutic services for those living with cancer. At the Healing Garden, she worked with people who faced unforgiving diagnoses. Her clients ranged from the newly diagnosed to those who were transitioning to end-of-life care in hospice. She witnessed the resilience of those who had suffered the unimaginable. Jacqueline is driven to help those who are vulnerable. Through her career, she has connected with people on a profound level, a place where few professionals ever have the privilege of entering.

www.ingramcontent.com/pod-product-compliance
Lightning Source LLC
Chambersburg PA
CBHW052028030426
42337CB00027B/4906